# MEN'S HEALTH: BODY, IDENTITY AND SOCIAL CONTEXT

Edited by

## Alex Broom PhD

*Senior Lecturer in Sociology, University of Newcastle, Australia*

## Philip Tovey PhD

*Reader in Health Sociology, University of Leeds, United Kingdom*

LIBRARIES WW RC

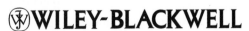

**WILEY-BLACKWELL**

A John Wiley & Sons, Ltd., Publication

**LIBRARIES NI**

C700144020

| | | |
|---|---|---|
| RONDO | 01/12/2009 | |
| 306.4613081 | £ 26.99 | |
| GENREF | | |

This edition first published 2009
© 2009 John Wiley & Sons, Ltd.

Wiley-Blackwell is an imprint of John Wiley & Sons, formed by the merger of
Wiley's global Scientific, Technical and Medical business with Blackwell
Publishing.

*Registered office*
John Wiley & Sons Ltd, The Atrium, Southern Gate, Chichester, West Sussex,
PO19 8SQ, United Kingdom

*Editorial office*
John Wiley & Sons Ltd, The Atrium, Southern Gate, Chichester, West Sussex,
PO19 8SQ, United Kingdom

For details of our global editorial offices, for customer services and for
information about how to apply for permission to reuse the copyright material in
this book please see our website at www.wiley.com/wiley-blackwell.

The right of the authors to be identified as the authors of this work has been
asserted in accordance with the Copyright, Designs and Patents Act 1988.

All rights reserved. No part of this publication may be reproduced, stored in a
retrieval system, or transmitted, in any form or by any means, electronic,
mechanical, photocopying, recording or otherwise, except as permitted by the
UK Copyright, Designs and Patents Act 1988, without the prior permission of
the publisher.

Wiley also publishes its books in a variety of electronic formats. Some content
that appears in print may not be available in electronic books.

Designations used by companies to distinguish their products are often claimed
as trademarks. All brand names and product names used in this book are trade
names, service marks, trademarks or registered trademarks of their respective
owners. The publisher is not associated with any product or vendor mentioned
in this book. This publication is designed to provide accurate and authoritative
information in regard to the subject matter covered. It is sold on the
understanding that the publisher is not engaged in rendering professional
services. If professional advice or other expert assistance is required, the services
of a competent professional should be sought.

*Library of Congress Cataloging-in-Publication Data*

Men's health : body, identity, and social context / edited by Alex Broom and
Philip Tovey.
        p. ; cm.
    Includes bibliographical references and index.
    ISBN 978-0-470-51656-0 (pbk. : alk. paper)    1. Men–Health and hygiene–Social
aspects.    2. Masculinity–Social aspects.    3. Body, Human–Social aspects.
4. Gender identity–Social aspects.    I. Broom, Alex.    II. Tovey, Philip, 1963-
    [DNLM:    1. Men's Health.    2. Gender Identity.    3. Health Behavior. WA
306 M548 2009]
    RA564.83.M49 2009
    362.1081–dc22
                                                                            2008032152

A catalogue record for this book is available from the British Library.

Set in 10/13.5 pt Trump Mediaeval by SNP Best-set Typesetter, Ltd., Hong Kong
Printed in Singapore by Markono Print Media Pte Ltd

1    2009

# CONTENTS

# CONTRIBUTORS

*Alex Broom*
Senior Lecturer in Sociology, University of Newcastle, Australia.

*Will Courtenay*
McLean Hospital, Harvard Medical School, USA.

*Mark Davis*
Lecturer in Sociology, School of Political and Social Inquiry, Faculty of
   Arts, Monash University, Australia.

*Richard de Visser*
Lecturer in Psychology, Department of Psychology, University of Sussex,
   United Kingdom.

*Paul M. Galdas*
Assistant Professor, School of Nursing, University of British Columbia,
   Canada.

*Julia Hall*
Associate Professor, D'Youville College, New York, USA.

*Helen Keane*
Senior Lecturer, College of Arts and Social Sciences, Australian National
   University, Australia.

*John L. Oliffe*
Associate Professor, School of Nursing, University of British Columbia,
   Canada.

*Bob Pease*
Professor of Social Work, School of Health & Social Development, Deakin University, Australia.

*Alan Petersen*
Professor of Sociology, Sociology Program, School of Political and Social Inquiry, Faculty of Arts, Monash University, Australia.

*Elianne Riska*
Professor of Sociology, Swedish School of Social Science, University of Helsinki, Finland.

*Don Sabo*
Professor of Sociology, Director, Center for Research on Physical Activity, Sport & Health, D'Youville College, New York, USA.

*Philip Tovey*
Reader in Health Sociology, University of Leeds, United Kingdom.

# INTRODUCTION: MEN'S HEALTH IN CONTEXT

Alex Broom and Philip Tovey

Research into men's health has proliferated in recent years with a focus on the ways in which gender constructions impact on men's health outcomes and everyday lives. Men's studies is now an established area within the social sciences with increasingly sophisticated theoretical and substantive work being produced internationally. We write this book at a time of emerging public and academic awareness of the adverse impacts of cultural enactments of masculinities on men and boys. From heart disease to mental illness and binge drinking, men's health is of increasing interest and concern to health policy-makers and healthcare practitioners. Despite this, health policy, public health campaigns and the focus of community health organisations are still strongly biased towards addressing women's health issues. In part, this is understandable, given the historical subordination of women and the negative influences of patriarchal dynamics on women's health and wellbeing; however, the result of ignoring the various difficulties posed by contemporary masculinities for men is a new type of gender gap that has wide-ranging implications.

This gender gap is perpetuated by the approaches of many healthcare practitioners and institutions, and is in turn legitimated through contemporary cultural beliefs around 'manliness' and (in)vulnerability. The result is a huge disparity in state funding and charity-based support for men's health as compared to women's health. Normative conceptions of hetero-masculinity lie at the core of the limited attention paid to men's health and wellbeing. Indeed, deeply embedded in the politics of gender and health is the assumption that men are in fact responsible for their ill health and that, if they actually asked for help, acted differently and got involved in health prevention, this gender gap would close. This is, at least in part, correct. So what is preventing men from doing these very things? As explored in the following chapters, the answer is both simple and highly complex. Contemporary masculinities, in their various forms, are at the

1

centre of this problematic of men's (ill) health. The seductivity of performing normative forms of heterosexual masculinity remains strong, and the
resulting health outcomes are often disastrous.

Suicide, depression, binge drinking, violence, heart disease and drug
taking: each is significantly higher among men than among women in
most western contexts and each is highly problematic for men's health
and wellbeing. While in some countries public health campaigns are emerging to address issues related to prostate cancer and depression, in reality
these attempts at public intervention promote very little in the way of
dialogue on the question of *why*. Rather, they merely attempt to *reform*
men's behaviour. Campaigns such as that on prostate cancer awareness,
for example, have attempted to *educate* men about risk and screening,
highlighting the benefits of early intervention. Few have even attempted
to address the systemic issues underlying cultural conceptions of masculine identity and their intersectionality with men's health and wellbeing.
For example, there is little public dialogue and debate about the cultural
problematic of the inability of *some* men to express weakness, discuss
vulnerability and reveal pain. Thus, while the underlying issues around
depression, late presentation of prostate cancer, suicide, excessive drinking
and so on are, albeit differentially, acknowledged as inextricably linked to
the enactment of masculine identities, there has been very little done in
the public sector to promote dialogue about culturally specific values
around 'manliness' that are involved in the production of these very health
problems. We are still faced with cultural stereotypes and narratives such
as 'men are bad with their health' without consideration of 'how society
is bad for men'. It is this very site of 'gender trouble' (Butler, 1990) which
critical masculinity studies, such as those presented in the following
chapters, seek to interrogate and reveal.

As shown in this book, the ways in which society can be 'bad for men'
are multiple and differentiated internationally; however, there are common
themes and consistencies that permeate each of the case studies examined.
What is clear, in these critical studies of masculinities, is that the ways
in which society is bad for men interplays with the very advantages that
some men have, thus making it difficult to disentangle disadvantage and
advantage. Indeed, such simplicities are inappropriate as a perceived site
of advantage may concurrently represent a site of disadvantage depending
on the actors involved and the specific sociocultural context. Here lies the
difficulty in engaging with the structural constraints and inequalities faced
by men; there is a historicity of structural constraint being inextricably
linked to 'maleness', thus problematising attempts to illustrate the ways
in which these very structures act in problematic ways on men. Some

concrete examples provide insight into such processes. High profile in the United Kingdom and Australia are the structural inequalities relating to men's access to their children after break-ups, the assumptions of courts in relation to mothering and fathering, and the inherent biases in the legal system in relation to men within family life. These social institutions and ideological positionings engender, reinforce and reproduce normative gender constructs and disadvantage men who attempt to challenge the prevailing orthodoxies of gender identity (in relation to parenting). The resulting mental health implications for men (and their families) are significant.

## Toward a new men's health

Some reflection on men's studies hitherto is useful at this point. Over-simplicity and lack of nuance in conceptions of 'men' and 'masculinity' plagued initial work in the area and has created unnecessary divisions with those working on women's health issues. There was (and to a certain extent still is) an element of 'protest' in the men's studies literature which has sought to redress the imbalance evident in the feminist-driven gender-and-health literature. While in some ways useful as a starting point for what is now a significant field of academic study, this early work in men's studies tended to reify monolithic conceptions of masculine identity, paying little or no attention to significant differentiation in masculinities according to ethnicity, sexuality, class, culture and so on. As such, 'masculine' was a monolithic conceptual device and was often conflated with ill health with little nuance expressed in terms of the intersectionality of masculinity identity and other facets of individual biography (Courtenay, 2000).

Raewyn Connell (1995), among others, encouraged a new emphasis in the men's studies literature, highlighting the limitations of non-differentiated conceptions of masculinity. Through reifying monolithic conceptions of masculinity, those working in the men's health field were in effect reinforcing the very categorical, binary-based inequalities they sought to address (Courtenay, 2000). There was a degree of complicity in the men's studies field in the production of divisive and non-differentiated conceptions of masculinity and health. Despite a new theoretical emphasis on *masculinities* (Connell, 1995), this did not substantially flow down to research in men's health for quite some time. In fact, while it was often acknowledged that masculinity was performative and multiple (i.e. it was shifting and 'a construct'), there were few substantive explorations into

the complex (and temporal) processes of masculine construction, enactment and resistance. This changed in the mid-1990s and particularly the
early 2000s with social science health researchers (including authors contributing to this text) increasingly exploring alternative, minority, protest
and marginalised masculinities, and how they interplay with various
health issues (e.g. Sabo & Gordon, 1995; Courtenay, 2000). Moreover,
social scientists began to provide thick descriptions and reflections on the
lived experiences of differently positioned men, illustrating the interplay
of masculinities and social life (including health), and providing a sense of
how men with diverse gender identities may experience such things as
surgery, cancer, depression, prostatic disease, heart disease, grief, decision
making and pain (e.g. Cameron & Bernardes, 1998; Chapple & Ziebland,
2002; Riska, 2002; Broom, 2004, 2005; Oliffe, 2005; Robertson,
2006).

Only in the last decade have health social scientists *begun* to understand
and represent the fluidity and multiplicity evident in the enactment of
masculine identities. A central component of new studies on men's health
has been their critical approach to masculinities, including an emphasis on
contingency and multiplicity. Moving from the binaries engendered in much
of the first wave of men's health research and writing, the emerging literature, often drawing on feminist theory, seeks to express a non-static, differentiated and temporal conceptualisation of contemporary masculinities.

Even with such progress in men's studies and despite the efforts of men's
health scholars to emphasise the importance of highlighting and addressing inequality emerging from conceptions of masculinity, such analyses
may be viewed by some as distracting from the wide-ranging implications
of gender 'ideals' for women, and thus, at least implicitly, reinforcing
patriarchal dynamics. While this is not true for significant proportions of
gender studies scholars, for a minority, the refocusing of gender and health
on men's health issues indicates a regression in work put into highlighting
the 'masculine' as dominator, rather than victim. In our view gender
studies should be the study of the impacts, enactments and implications
of gender ideals, not the pursuit of the negative implications of gender for
women. Furthermore, and although rather simplistically, there are certain
benefits for women resulting from the enactment of idealised gender constructs. In saying this, it is crucial that men's studies scholars also contribute to the implications of various constructions of masculinity for
women; conceptualising victim status will do little to create dialogue and
constructive conversations.

Ultimately the work done by those working in men's health *is* compat-
ible with that which has been done and continues to be done in gender

studies and women's health research. The emphasis on the 'troubles' with masculinities, for men, further captures the restrictive components of gender ideals for both men and women. There will, inevitably, always be some resistance within gender studies circles to acknowledging the plight of men; just as there will be stalwarts in the men's health movement who give too little attention to the ongoing structural inequalities shaping women's experiences of health within the context of restrictive gender dynamics. Here we push past such restrictive perspectives, focusing on understanding the complexities of gender-identity enactment, the inter-sectionality of gender, ethnicity, class and age, and the specificity of iden-tity to cultural and historical context.

In this book we have drawn together academics at the forefront of research into men's health, each examining a different site of 'trouble' and enactment of masculinity, and the implications for men's health and wellbeing. In selecting these authors we aimed to provide an international and interdis-ciplinary perspective on the state of play in men's health research. Including authors from the United States, United Kingdom, Canada, Finland and Aus-tralia, we have brought together a diverse set of studies from a variety of cultural contexts to interrogate the ways in which masculinity is performed, enacted, resisted and constructed. All utilise a critical social science perspec-tive, drawing on a range of disciplinary backgrounds and methodologies to tease out key issues. Moreover, in selecting a diverse range of topics (from prostate cancer and heart disease to sport) we aimed to bring together a range of bodily contexts and cultural forums.

Our approach to editing these chapters was to allow the authors to maintain their own conceptual lens, rather than imposing a strict model of masculinity or of gender and health. For that reason, this collection does not represent a set of papers that are, ultimately, in complete agreement; rather, although consistent in their critical approaches and overall agenda (i.e. to identify and interrogate gendered dynamics which impact on men's health and wellbeing), each has its own particular bent on the theoretical strengths within existing literature, substantive gaps, and the area where men's studies should move from here. As such, they should be read as individual pieces within an overall framework designed to provide a coher-ent sense of the state of play in men's health internationally.

## Outline of the book

We begin with a chapter by Will Courtenay providing a theoretical and substantive overview of men's health, drawing on a range of theoretical perspectives to critically examine the ways in which researchers and academics have engaged with the area. Will Courtenay's chapter outlines a comprehensive theory of masculinity and health, which is ultimately progressive rather than divisive in character. This sets up the following chapters which examine specific substantive issues of concern in contemporary studies of men's health and masculinities.

In Chapter 2, engaging with the contemporary experience of prostate cancer, John Oliffe contributes a photo-elicitation/qualitative interview study, exploring men's experiences of prostate cancer and the interplay of impotence, incontinence and various prostatic procedures on men's gender identities. A key strength of this chapter is its engagement with the temporality of disease experience, including the complex implications of prostatic disease for gender identities before, during and after treatment. This is an unusual and revealing methodological approach, involving analysis of self-representation (photos) and interactive dialogue (interviews) to trace the significant complexity in men's narratives of disease.

A classic argument in the men's health literature has been the so-called resistance of men to seek help, and the implications for men's health and disease mortality. In Chapter 3, Paul Galdas examines the highly complex and culturally differentiated issue of help-seeking, critically exploring the stereotypical cultural conception of men as 'bad' help-seekers. Continuing the critical approach to masculinities seen in the previous two chapters, this analysis emphasises the intersectionality of ethnicity, race and sexuality in help-seeking, espousing a more situated and temporal view of contemporary masculinities, and focusing on developing a more progressive and less monolithic conceptual lens for understanding help-seeking behaviours.

While the previous chapters analyse men's narratives of health and illness, in Chapter 4, Don Sabo and Julia Hall draw together the accounts of both men *and* women to explore the gendered nature of experiences of heart disease. Utilising a relational approach to examining the interplay of gender and health, they critically examine experiences of coronary heart disease in the US, illustrating the intersectionality of race, class and gender in shaping individuals' experiences of disease. They develop a temporal conceptualisation of gendered disease experience as ultimately relational as evidenced in men's and women's lived experiences.

In Chapter 5, Mark Davis draws sexuality into the mix, engaging with the interplay of masculinities, sexualities, disease and virtuality. In an intriguing and novel analysis of spectacular risk in the context of marginalised masculinities, Mark examines HIV risk-taking behaviour among gay men and, specifically, 'barebacking' as a cultural phenomenon. Critiquing previous representations of barebacking and links to normative conceptions of 'risky' masculinities, this chapter develops a nuanced discussion of sexual practice within the gay community, deconstructing the 'spectacle' of barebacking and critiquing social scientists' simplistic conceptions of risk.

Our sixth chapter, by Richard de Visser, examines binge drinking as seen in everyday lives of young British men. This chapter utilises both quantitative and qualitative data to illustrate the intersectionality of culture, gender and alcohol consumption. In a sociocultural context in which 'binge drinking' is high on the British political agenda (including law reform and public health interventions), this chapter posits a more nuanced and less linear conception of alcohol and masculinity, emphasising both the problematic of binge-drinking cultures as well as the ambivalence of some young men to alcohol and sites of resistance.

On a related area, in Chapter 7, Elianne Riska examines the state of play in men's mental health research and the theoretical underpinnings of existing work in the area of mental health and gender. This is a particularly valuable contribution as it engages with an area that has been hugely undertheorised, exploring the evolution and often misguided nature of mental health theoretical models. This chapter unpacks the historical and assumptive underpinnings of much mental health research and theorising, tracing, among other things, the 'gendering' of psychological conditions and symptomatology.

Moving toward a focus on culture and gender performativity, in Chapter 8 Helen Keane examines bodybuilding as a form of ethical self-formation rather than merely an enactment of hegemonic masculinities. Bodybuilding has historically been presented as a rather pathological site of hypermasculine expression, with critique focused on, among other things, the idealisation of muscular/aggressive masculinities. In a fascinating departure from traditional analyses of sport and masculinities, this chapter deconstructs 'building the body' as dysfunction, examining how the 'players' themselves present their activities. Offering fascinating insight into the paradoxes between sport and health, this chapter delves into men's grassroots narratives of health and harm, self-discipline and self-formation, within a unique sporting subculture.

In Chapter 9, the final empirical chapter, we see race and ethnicity as they interplay with masculinities in contemporary Australian society. In particular, Bob Pease looks at the intersectionality of race and ethnicity with masculinity, focusing on the experiences of refugees and immigrant men in Australia. This chapter illustrates how masculinities, in interaction with racial and ethnic identification and social class, create particular health risks for men. This is a particularly useful contribution given that very little research on men's health has explored the experiences of immigrant and refugee men, and furthermore, little research on migrant and refugee health has explored the roles of masculinities. Drawing on feminist intersectional analysis, critical masculinity studies and critical race theory, this chapter inserts a new layer of complexity into the debate over men's health outcomes.

In the final chapter to this collection, Alan Petersen outlines a future research agenda in men's health. In particular he focuses on the importance of continuing the work being done in men's health to transcend essentialism, dualistic models of gender and health, and oversimplistic power-based conceptions of gender-based patriarchy and oppression. This chapter provides a valuable reminder to those developing research programmes in men's health of the mistakes of the past and the challenges and potential for the future.

# References

Broom, A. (2004) Prostate cancer and masculinity in Australian society: a case of stolen identity? *International Journal of Men's Health*, **3**(2), 73–91.

Broom, A. (2005) The eMale: prostate cancer, masculinity and online support as a challenge to medical expertise. *Journal of Sociology*, **41**(1), 87–104.

Butler, J. (1990) *Gender Trouble: Feminism and the Subversion of Identity*. New York: Routledge.

Cameron, E. & Bernardes, J. (1998) Gender and disadvantage in health: men's health for a change. *Sociology of Health and Illness*, **20**(5), 673–693.

Chapple, A. & Ziebland, S. (2002) Prostate cancer: embodied experience and perceptions of masculinity. *Sociology of Health and Illness*, **24**(6), 820–841.

Connell, R.W. (1995) *Masculinities*. Sydney: Allen & Unwin.

Courtenay, W.H. (2000) Constructions of masculinity and their influence on men's well-being: a theory of gender and health. *Social Science and Medicine*, **50**(10), 1385–1401.

Oliffe, J.L. (2005) Constructions of masculinity following prostatectomy-induced impotence. *Social Science and Medicine*, **60**(10), 2240–2259.

Riska, E. (2002) From type A man to the hardy man: masculinity and health. *Sociology of Health and Illness*, **24**(3), 347–358.

Robertson, S. (2006) 'I've been like a coiled spring this last week': embodied masculinity and health. *Sociology of Health & Illness* **28**(4), 433–456.

Sabo, D. & Gordon, D.F. (1995) *Men's Health and Illness: Gender, Power and the Body*. Thousand Oaks, CA: Sage Publications.

# Chapter 1

# THEORISING MASCULINITY AND MEN'S HEALTH

Will Courtenay

## Introduction

Men in the United States, on average, die more than 5 years younger than women (Department of Health and Human Services [DHHS], 2007). For all 15 leading causes of death, except Alzheimer's disease, and in every age group, men and boys have higher death rates than women and girls (Courtenay, 2003). Men's age-adjusted death rate for heart disease and cancer are both 1.5 times higher than women's (DHHS, 2007). Men are also more likely than women to suffer severe chronic conditions and fatal diseases (Verbrugge & Wingard, 1987), and to suffer them at an earlier age. Nearly three out of four persons who die from heart attacks before age 65 are men (American Heart Association, 1995). Similar patterns in morbidity and mortality have been observed in the UK, Canada and Australia (see Courtenay, 2002; and Chapters 3, 6 and 9).

A variety of factors influence and are associated with health and longevity, including economic status, ethnicity, and access to care (Laveist, 1993; Pappas et al., 1993; Doyal, 1995). However, these factors cannot explain gender differences in health and longevity. For instance, while lack of adequate healthcare, poor nutrition and substandard housing all contribute to the health problems of African Americans (Gibbs, 1988), they cannot account for cancer death rates that are nearly twice as high among African American men than among African American women (American Cancer Society, 2005). Health behaviours, however, do help to explain gender differences in health and longevity. An independent scientific panel established by the US government has evaluated thousands of research studies and estimated that half of all deaths in the US could be prevented through changes in personal health practices (US Preventive Services Task Force [USPSTF], 1996). Similar conclusions have been reached by other health experts reviewing hundreds of studies (Woolf et al., 1996).

Gender is one of the most important sociocultural factors associated with and influencing health-related behaviour. Women engage in far more health-promoting behaviours than men and have more healthy lifestyle patterns (see Courtenay, 2000a). Being a woman may, in fact, be the strongest predictor of preventive and health-promoting behaviour (see Courtenay, 2000a). A recent, extensive review of large studies, national data and metanalyses summarises evidence of sex differences in behaviours that significantly influence health and longevity (Courtenay, 2000a). This review systematically demonstrates that males of all ages are more likely than females to engage in over 30 behaviours that increase the risk of disease, injury and death. This gender difference in health behaviours remains true across a variety of racial and ethnic groups (Courtenay et al., 2002).

Findings are generally similar for healthcare visits. Although gender differences in utilisation generally begin to disappear when the health problem is more serious (Verbrugge, 1985; Waldron, 1988; Mor et al., 1990), adult men make far fewer healthcare visits than women do, independent of reproductive healthcare visits (Verbrugge, 1985, 1988; Kandrack et al., 1991). According to the US Department of Health and Human Services (1998), among persons *with health problems*, men are significantly more likely than women to have had no recent physician contacts, regardless of income or ethnicity; poor men are twice as likely as poor women to have had no recent contact, and high-income men are two and a half times as likely as high-income women.

Despite their enormous health effects, few researchers or theorists have offered explanations for these gender differences in behaviour, or for their implications for men's health (Verbrugge, 1985; Sabo & Gordon, 1995; Courtenay, 1998a, 2000b, 2002; Courtenay & Keeling, 2000a, b). Although health science of this century has frequently used males as study subjects, research typically neglects to examine men and the health risks associated with men's gender. Little is known about *why* men engage in less healthy lifestyles and adopt fewer health-promoting beliefs and behaviours. The health risks associated with men's gender or masculinity have remained largely unproblematic and taken for granted. The consistent, underlying presumption in medical literature is that what it means to be a man in America has no bearing on how men work, drink, drive, fight or take risks. Left unquestioned, men's shorter lifespan is often presumed to be natural and inevitable.

This paper proposes a relational theory of men's health from a social constructionist and feminist perspective. It provides an introduction to social constructionist perspectives on gender and a brief critique of gender role theory before illustrating how health beliefs and behaviour are used in constructing gender in North America, and how masculinity and health are constructed within a relational context. It further examines how men construct various forms of masculinity – or masculinities – and how these different enactments of gender, as well as differing social structural influences, contribute to differential health risks among men in the US.

## Health and the social construction of gender

### Constructionism and theories of gender

Previous explanations of masculinity and men's health have focused primarily on the hazardous influences of *'the* male sex role' (Goldberg, 1976; Nathanson, 1977; Harrison, 1978; Verbrugge, 1985; Harrison et al., 1992). These explanations relied on theories of gender socialisation that have since been widely criticised (Deaux, 1984; Gerson & Peiss, 1985; Kimmel, 1986; Pleck, 1987; West & Zimmerman, 1987; Epstein, 1988; Messerschmidt, 1993; Connell, 1995). The sex role theory of socialisation, for example, has been criticised for implying that gender represents 'two fixed, static, and mutually exclusive role containers' (Kimmel, 1986, p.521) and for assuming that women and men have innate psychological needs for gender-stereotypic traits (Pleck, 1987). Sex role theory also fosters the notion of a singular female or male personality, a notion that has been effectively disputed, and obscures the various forms of femininity and masculinity that women and men can and do demonstrate (Connell, 1995).

From a constructionist perspective, women and men think and act in the ways that they do, not because of their role identities or psychological traits, but because of concepts about femininity and masculinity that they adopt from their culture (Pleck et al., 1994a). Gender is not two static categories, but rather 'a set of socially constructed relationships which are produced and reproduced through people's actions' (Gerson & Peiss, 1985, p.327); it is constructed by dynamic, dialectic relationships (Connell, 1995). Gender is 'something that one does, and *does* recurrently, in interaction with others' (West & Zimmerman, 1987, p.140); it is achieved or demonstrated and is better understood as a verb than as a noun (Kaschak, 1992; Bohan, 1993; Crawford, 1995). Most importantly, gender does not reside in the person, but rather in social transactions defined as gendered (Bohan, 1993; Crawford, 1995). From this perspective, gender is viewed as a dynamic, social structure.

## Gender stereotypes

Gender is constructed from cultural and subjective meanings that constantly shift and vary, depending on the time and place. Gender stereotypes are among the meanings used by society in the construction of gender, and are characteristics that are generally believed to be typical either of women or of men. There is very high agreement in our society about what are considered to be typically feminine and typically masculine characteristics (Williams & Best, 1990; Golombok & Fivush, 1994; Street et al., 1995). These stereotypes provide collective, organised – and dichotomous – meanings of gender and often become widely shared beliefs about who women and men innately *are* (Pleck, 1987). People are encouraged to conform to stereotypic beliefs and behaviours, and commonly do conform to and adopt dominant norms of femininity and masculinity (Eagly, 1983; Deaux, 1984; Bohan, 1993). Conforming to what is expected of them further reinforces self-fulfilling prophecies of such behaviour (Geis, 1993; Crawford, 1995).

Research indicates that men and boys experience comparatively greater social pressure than women and girls to endorse gendered societal prescriptions – such as the strongly endorsed *health-related* beliefs that men are independent, self-reliant, strong, robust and tough (Williams & Best, 1990; Golombok & Fivush, 1994; Martin, 1995). It is, therefore, not surprising that their behaviour and their beliefs about gender are more stereotypic than those of women and girls (Katz & Ksansnak, 1994; Rice & Coates, 1995; Street et al., 1995; Levant & Majors, 1998). From a social constructionist perspective, however, men and boys are not passive victims of a socially prescribed role, nor are they simply conditioned or socialised by their cultural context. Men and boys are active agents in constructing and reconstructing dominant norms of masculinity. This concept of agency – the part individuals play in exerting power and producing effects in their lives – is central to constructionism (Courtenay, 2000b).

## Health beliefs and behaviours: resources for constructing gender

The activities that men and women engage in, and their gendered cognitions, are a form of currency in transactions that are continually enacted in the demonstration of gender. Previous authors have examined how a variety of activities are used as resources in constructing and reconstructing gender; these activities include language (Perry et al., 1992; Crawford, 1995), work (Connell, 1995), sports (Connell, 1992; Messner & Sabo, 1994), crime (Messerschmidt, 1993) and sex (Vance, 1995). The very manner in which women and men carry out these activities contributes both to the defining of one's self as gendered and to social conventions of gender.

Health-related beliefs and behaviours can similarly be understood as a means of constructing or demonstrating gender (see Courtenay, 2000b). In this way, the health behaviours and beliefs that people adopt simultaneously define and enact representations of gender. Health beliefs and behaviours, like language, can be understood as 'a set of strategies for negotiating the social landscape' (Crawford, 1995, p.17), or tools for constructing gender. Like crime, health behaviour 'may be invoked as a practice through which masculinities (and men and women) are differentiated from one another' (Messerschmidt, 1993, p.85). The findings from one small study examining gender differences and health led the author to conclude that 'the doing of health is a form of doing gender' (Saltonstall, 1993, p.12). In this regard, 'health actions are social acts' and 'can be seen as a form of practice which constructs . . . "the person" in the same way that other social and cultural activities do' (Saltonstall, 1993, p.12).

The social experiences of women and men provide a template that guides their beliefs and behaviour. The various social transactions, institutional structures and contexts that women and men encounter elicit different demonstrations of health beliefs and behaviours, and provide different opportunities to conduct this particular form of demonstrating gender. If these social experiences and demonstrated beliefs or behaviours had no bearing on the health of women and men, they would be of no relevance here. This, however, is not the case. The social practices required for demonstrating femininity and masculinity are associated with very different health advantages and risks (Courtenay, 2000b). Unlike the presumably innocent effects of wearing lipstick or wearing a tie, the use of health-related beliefs and behaviours to define oneself as a woman or a man has a profound impact on one's health and longevity.

## Theorising masculinity in the context of health

The following sections provide a relational analysis of men's gendered health behaviour based on constructionist and feminist theories, and examine how cultural dictates, everyday interactions and social and institutional structures help to sustain and reproduce men's health risks.

### Gender, power, and the social construction of the 'stronger' sex

A discussion of power and social inequality is necessary to understand the broader context of men's adoption of unhealthy behaviour – as well as to address the social structures that both foster unhealthy behaviour among men and undermine men's attempts to adopt healthier habits. Gender is negotiated in part through relationships of power. Micro-level power practices (Pyke, 1996) contribute to structuring the social transactions of everyday life, transactions that help to sustain and reproduce broader structures of power and inequality. These power relationships are located in and constituted in, among other practices, the practice of health behaviour. The systematic subordination of women and lower-status men – or patriarchy – is made possible, in part, through these gendered demonstrations of health and health behaviour. In this way, males use health beliefs and behaviours to demonstrate dominant – and hegemonic – masculine ideals that clearly establish them as men. Hegemonic masculinity is the idealised form of masculinity at a given place and time (Connell, 1995). It is the socially dominant gender construction that subordinates femininities as well as other forms of masculinity, and reflects and shapes men's social relationships with women and other men; it represents power and authority. Today in the US, hegemonic masculinity is embodied in heterosexual, highly educated, European American men of upper-class economic status.

The fact that there are a variety of health risks associated with being a man in no way implies that men do not hold power. Indeed, it is in the pursuit of power and privilege that men are often led to harm themselves (Clatterbaugh, 1997). The social practices that undermine men's health are often the instruments men use in the structuring and acquisition of power. Men's acquisition of power requires, for example, that men suppress their needs and refuse to admit to or acknowledge their pain (Kaufman, 1994). Additional health-related beliefs and behaviours that can be used in the demonstration of hegemonic masculinity include the denial of weakness or vulnerability, emotional and physical control, the appearance of being strong and robust, dismissal of any need for help, a ceaseless interest in sex, the display of aggressive behaviour, and physical dominance. These health-related demonstrations of gender and power represent forms of micro-level power practices, practices that are 'part of a system that affirms and (re)constitutes broader relations of inequality' (Pyke, 1996, p.546). In exhibiting or enacting hegemonic ideals with health behaviours, men reinforce strongly held cultural beliefs that men are more powerful and less vulnerable than women; that men's bodies are structurally more efficient than and superior to women's bodies; that asking for help and caring for one's health are feminine; and that the most powerful men among men are those for whom health and safety are irrelevant.

It has been demonstrated elsewhere (Courtenay, 1998a, 1999, 2000b) that the resources available in the US for constructing masculinities are largely unhealthy. Men and boys often use these resources and reject healthy beliefs and behaviours in order to demonstrate and achieve manhood. By dismissing their healthcare needs, men are constructing gender. When a man brags, 'I haven't been to a doctor in years,' he is simultaneously describing a health practice and situating himself in a masculine arena. Similarly, men are demonstrating dominant norms of masculinity when they refuse to take sick leave from work, when they insist that they need little sleep, and when they boast that drinking does not impair their driving. Men also construct masculinities by embracing risk. A man may define the degree of his masculinity, for example, by driving dangerously or performing risky sports – and displaying these behaviours like badges of honour. In these ways, and as shown in the following chapters, masculinities are defined *against* positive health behaviours and beliefs.

To carry out any one positive health behaviour, a man may need to reject multiple constructions of masculinity. For example, the application of sunscreen to prevent skin cancer – the most rapidly increasing cancer in the US (Centers for Disease Control [CDC], 1995a) – may require the rejection of a variety of social constructions: masculine men are unconcerned about health matters; masculine men are invulnerable to disease; the application of lotions to the body is a feminine pastime; masculine men don't 'pamper' or 'fuss' over their bodies; and 'rugged good looks' are produced with a tan. In *not* applying sunscreen, a man may be simultaneously demonstrating gender and an unhealthy practice. The facts that 1.5 times more men than women nationally believe that one looks better with a tan (American Academy of Dermatology, 1997), that men are significantly less likely to use sunscreen (Mermelstein & Riesenberg, 1992; Courtenay 1998a, b), and that the skin cancer death rate is twice as high for men as for women (CDC, 1995b), may be a testament to the level of support among men for endorsing these constructions.

When a man does experience an illness or disability, the gender ramifications are often great. Illness 'can reduce a man's status in masculine hierarchies, shift his power relations with women, and raise his self-doubts about masculinity' (Charmaz, 1995, p.268). The friend of a US senator cautioned him against publicly discussing his diagnosis of prostate cancer, contending that 'some men might see [his] willingness to go public with his private struggle as a sign of weakness' (Jaffe, 1997, p.134). In efforts to preserve their masculinity, one researcher found that men with chronic illnesses often worked diligently to hide their disabilities: a man with diabetes, unable to manoeuvre both his wheelchair and a cafeteria tray, would skip lunch and risk a coma rather than request assistance; a middle-aged man declined offers of easier jobs to prove that he was still capable of strenuous work; an executive concealed dialysis treatments by telling others that he was away attending meetings (Charmaz, 1995).

### Feminities and men's health

It is not only the endorsement of hegemonic ideals but also the rejection of feminine ideals that contributes to the construction of masculinities and to the systematic oppression of women and less powerful men. Rejecting what is constructed as feminine is essential for demonstrating hegemonic masculinity in a sexist and gender-dichotomous society. Men and boys who attempt to engage in social action that demonstrates feminine norms of gender, risk being relegated to the subordinated masculinity of 'wimp' or 'sissy'. Healthcare utilisation and positive health beliefs or behaviours are also socially constructed as forms of idealised femininity (Courtenay, 1999, 2000b, 2004a, b). They are, therefore, potentially feminising influences that men must oppose with varying degrees of force, depending on what other resources are accessible or are being utilised in the construction of masculinities. Forgoing healthcare is a means of rejecting 'girl stuff'.

Men's risk-taking, and denial and disregard of physical discomfort and healthcare needs, are all means of demonstrating difference from women, who are presumed to embody these 'feminine' characteristics. These behaviours serve both as proof of men's superiority over women and as proof of their ranking among 'real' men. A man's success in adopting (socially feminised) health-promoting behaviour, like his failure to engage in (socially masculinised) physically risky behaviour, can undermine his ranking among men and relegate him to a subordinated status. That men and boys construct masculinities in opposition to the healthy beliefs and behaviours of women – and less masculine (i.e. 'feminised') men and boys – is clearly apparent in their discourse, as evidenced by the remarks of one firefighter: 'When you go out to fires, you will work yourself into the ground. Just so nobody else thinks you're a puss' (Delsohn, 1996, p.95). In prison, men criticise fellow prisoners who 'complain too much' about sickness or pain or make frequent healthcare visits, as displaying signs of 'softness' (Courtenay & Sabo, 2001).

### Differences among men

Contemporary feminist theorists are as concerned about differences among men (and among women) as they are about differences between women and men. As Messerschmidt (1993, p.87) notes, '"Boys will be boys" differently, depending upon their position in social structures and, there-fore, upon their access to power and resources.' Although men may endorse similar masculine ideals, different men may enact these ideals in different ways. For example, although most young men in the US may agree that a man should be 'tough' (Courtenay, 1998a), *how* each man demonstrates being tough – and how demonstrating toughness affects him physically – will be influenced by his age, ethnicity, social class and sexuality. Depend-ing upon these factors, a man may use a gun, his fists, his sexuality, a mountain bike, physical labour, a car or the relentless pursuit of financial strength to construct this particular aspect of masculinity.

Social class positioning 'both constrains and enables certain forms of gendered social action' (Messerschmidt, 1993, p.94) and influences which unhealthy behaviours are used to demonstrate masculinity. Demonstrating masculinities with fearless, high-risk behaviours may entail skydiving for an upper-class man, mountain climbing for a middle-class man, racing hot rods for a working-class man, and street fighting for a poor urban man. Many working-class masculinities that are constructed as exemplary – as in the case of firemen – require the dismissal of fear, and feats of physical endur-ance and strength, that often put these men at risk of injury and death. The avoidance of healthcare is another form of social action that allows some men to maintain their status and to avoid being relegated to a subordinated position in relation to physicians and health professionals, as well as other men. For an upper-middle-class business executive, refusing to see a physi-cian can be a means of maintaining his position of power.

The construction of health and gender does not occur in isolation from other forms of social action that demonstrate differences among men. Health practices may be used simultaneously to enact multiple social constructions, such as ethnicity, class and sexuality. The use of health beliefs and behaviours to construct the interacting social structures of masculinity and ethnicity is illustrated in this passage by a Chicano novelist:

> *A macho doesn't show weakness. Grit your teeth, take the pain, bear it alone. Be tough. You feel like letting it out! Well, then let's get drunk with our compadres . . . Drinking buddies who have a contest to see who can consume the most beer, or the most shots of tequila, are trying to prove their maleness.* (Anaya, 1996, p.63)

Too often, factors such as ethnicity, class, and sexuality are simply treated by health scientists as variables to be controlled for in statistical analyses. However, the social structuring of ethnicity, sexuality and class is intima-tely and systematically related to the social structuring of gender and power (see Courtenay, 2001a, 2002). These various social structures are constructed concurrently and are intertwined. When European American working-class boys speed recklessly through a poor African American neighbourhood, not wearing safety belts and yelling epithets out their windows, they are using health risk behaviours – among other behaviours – in the simultaneous construction of gender, power, class and ethnicity; when they continue these behaviours in a nearby gay neighbourhood, they are further reproducing gender, power and normative heterosexuality. Similarly, poor health beliefs and behaviours are used by men and boys to construct masculinities in conjunction with the use of other behaviours such as crime (Messerschmidt, 1993), work (Pyke, 1996) and being 'cool' (Majors & Billson, 1992). Committing criminal acts may be insufficient to win a young man inclusion in a street gang; he may also be required to prove his manhood by demonstrating his willingness to ignore pain or to engage in physical fighting.

## Making a difference: the negotiation of power and status

Just as men exercise varying degrees of power over women, so they exercise varying degrees of power among themselves. 'Masculinities are configurations of social practices produced not only in relation to femininities but also in relation to one another' (Pyke, 1996, p.531). Dominant masculinities subordinate lower-status, marginalised masculinities – such as those of gay, rural or lower-class men (Courtenay & Sabo, 2001; Courtenay, 2002, 2006). In negotiating this perilous landscape of masculinities, the male body is often used as a vehicle. The comments of one man in prison illustrate how the male body can be used in structuring gender and power:

> I have been shot and stabbed. Each time I wore bandages like a badge of honor . . . Each situation made me feel a little more tougher than the next guy . . . Being that I had survived, these things made me feel bigger because I could imagine that the average person couldn't go through a shoot out or a knife fight, survive and get right back into the action like it was nothing. The perception that I had constructed in my mind was that most people were discouraged after almost facing death, but the really bad ones could look death in the eye with little or no compunction. (Courtenay & Sabo, 2001, p.161)

Physical dominance and violence are easily accessible resources for structuring, negotiating and sustaining masculinities, particularly among men who because of their social positioning lack less dangerous means.

The health risks associated with any form of masculinity will differ depending on whether a man is enacting a hegemonic, subordinated, marginalised, complicit or resistant form. When men and boys are denied access to the social power and resources necessary for constructing hegemonic masculinity, they must seek other resources for constructing gender that validate their masculinity (Messerschmidt, 1993). Disadvantages resulting from such factors as ethnicity, class, educational level and sexual orientation marginalise certain men and augment the relevance of enacting other forms of masculinity. Rejecting health behaviours that are socially constructed as feminine, embracing risk and demonstrating fearlessness are readily accessible means of enacting masculinity. As one young man reported, 'If somebody picks on you or something, and you don't fight back, they'll call you a chicken. But . . . if you fight back . . . you're cool' (Majors & Billson 1992, p.26). Among some African American men and boys, 'toughness, violence, and disregard of death and danger become the hallmark of survival in a world that does not respond to reasonable efforts to belong and achieve' (Majors & Billson, 1992, p.34). The results of one small study suggest that toughness and aggression are indeed means for young inner-city African American men to gain status in communities where few other means of doing so are available: 'If a young man is a "tough guy," peers respect him . . . The highest value is placed on individuals who defend themselves swiftly, even if by doing so they place themselves in danger' (Rich & Stone, 1996, p.81).

Marginalised men may also attempt to compensate for their subordinated status by defying hegemonic masculinity and constructing alternative forms of masculinity. As Pyke (1996, p.531) explains, men 'with their masculine identity and self-esteem undermined by their subordinate order-taking position in relation to higher-status males' can and do use other resources to 'reconstruct their position as embodying *true* masculinity' (emphasis added). Other authors have variously referred to these alternative enactments of gender as *oppositional* (Messerschmidt, 1993), *compulsive* (Majors & Billson, 1992), *compensatory* (Pyke, 1996), or *protest* (Connell, 1995) masculinities. These 'hypermasculine' constructions are frequently dangerous or self-destructive (Meinecke, 1981). Majors and Billson (1992, p.34) suggest that compulsive masculinity can 'lead toward smoking, drug and alcohol abuse, fighting, sexual conquests, dominance, and crime'. Pyke (1996, p.538) describes lower-class men who 'ostentatiously pursued drugs, alcohol, and sexual carousing . . . [to compensate] for their subordinated status in the hierarchy of their everyday work worlds'. Similarly, working-class men can and do 'use the physical endurance and tolerance of discomfort required of their manual labor as signifying true masculinity, [as] an alternative to the hegemonic form' (Pyke, 1996, p.531). When the demonstration of the (dominant) heterosexist ideal is not an option – as among gay men – dismissing the risks associated with high numbers of sexual partners or unprotected anal intercourse can serve for some men as a means of demonstrating a protest masculinity. In describing coming out gay, one young man said, 'Rage, rage, rage! Let's do everything you've denied yourself for 25 years. Let's get into it and have a good time sexually' (Connell, 1995, p.153).

Like unhealthy behaviours, dominant or idealised beliefs or attitudes about manhood also provide the means for demonstrating gender. These signifiers of 'true' masculinity are readily accessible to men who may otherwise have limited social resources for constructing masculinity. In fact, among young men nationally, lower educational level, lower family income and African American ethnicity are all associated with traditional, dominant norms of masculinity (Courtenay, 1998a). The stronger endorsement of traditional masculine ideology among African American men than among non-African American men is a consistent finding (Pleck et al., 1994b; Levant & Majors, 1998; Levant et al., 1998). Among African American men, the endorsement of dominant norms of masculinity is stronger for both younger and non-professional men than it is for older, professional men (Hunter & Davis, 1992; Harris et al., 1994). Similarly, national data indicate that young men in the US who are not exclusively heterosexual hold more traditional or dominant beliefs about masculinity than young men who are exclusively heterosexual (Courtenay, 1998a). The endorsement of hypermasculine beliefs can be understood as a means for gay and bisexual men to prove to others that, despite their sexual preferences, they are still 'real' men.

A growing body of research provides evidence that men who endorse dominant norms of masculinity engage in poorer health behaviours and have greater health risks than their peers with less traditional beliefs (see Courtenay, 2003 for a review; Courtenay & McCreary, in press). One longitudinal study of 1,676 young men in the US, aged 15 to 23 years, is among the few nationally representative studies to examine the influence of masculinity on health behaviour over time. When a variety of psychosocial factors were controlled for, beliefs about masculinity emerged as the strongest predictor of risk-taking behaviour 2.5 years later (Courtenay, 1998a). Dominant norms of masculinity – the most traditional beliefs about manhood adopted by young men – predicted the highest level of risk-taking and of involvement in behaviours such as cigarette smoking, high-risk sexual activity and use of alcohol and other drugs.

## Rethinking compulsive, oppositional, compensatory, and protest masculinities

The terms *compulsive, oppositional, compensatory* and *protest* masculinities can be somewhat misleading. *Most* men are compulsive in demonstrating masculinity, which, as Connell (1995) notes, is continually contested. Furthermore, *most* masculinities that men demonstrate in the US are oppositional or compensatory; relatively few men construct the hegemonic masculine ideal. This is not to suggest, however, that hegemonic masculinity is not profoundly influential. On the contrary, hegemonic masculinity is a ubiquitous aspect of North American life. Most men necessarily demonstrate alternative masculinities in relation to hegemonic masculinity that variously aspire to, conspire with, or attempt to resist, diminish or otherwise undermine hegemonic masculinity. They do this not only in relation to other men perceived to embody hegemonic ideals, but also in relation to institutionalised, hegemonic social structures – including the government and media, the judicial system, corporate and technological industries, and academia. However, to suggest that only certain men are compulsive in demonstrating dominant norms of masculinity is to risk further marginalising the subordinated masculinities of lower-class, non-European American, non-heterosexual men. Masculinity *requires* compulsive practice, because it can be contested and undermined at any moment.

## Further contextualising men's health

As Messerschmidt (1993, p.83) notes, 'Although men attempt to express hegemonic masculinity through speech, dress, physical appearance, activities, and relations with others, these social signs of masculinity are associated with the specific context of one's actions and are self-regulated within that context.' Because masculinity is continually contested, it must be renegotiated in each context that a man encounters. A man or boy will enact gender and health differently in different contexts. On the football field, a college student may use exposure to injury and denial of pain to demonstrate masculinity, while at parties he may use excessive drinking to achieve the same end. A man may consider the expression of emotional or physical pain to be unacceptable with other men, but acceptable with a spouse or girlfriend. In some contexts, such as a prison setting (Courtenay & Sabo, 2001), the hierarchies of masculinities are unique to that particular context.

Farm life provides a context within which to examine the negotiation of one form of rural masculinity. Growing up on a farm, much of what boys learn to do to demonstrate hegemonic masculinity requires them to adopt risky or unhealthy behaviours, such as operating heavy equipment before they are old enough to do so safely (for an extensive discussion, see Courtenay, 2006). As two rural men said, 'If you're over ten, you'd better be out doing men's work, driving a tractor and that kind of thing' (Fellows, 1996, p.173); 'My brother Tony and I started driving the pickup on the farm at age six, as soon as we could reach the pedals. We also learned how to drive a tractor' (Fellows, 1996, p.305). The ways to enact masculinity are dictated in part by cultural norms, such as the belief held by most Pennsylvanians that 'farmers *embody* the virtues of independence and self-sufficiency' (Willits et al., 1990, p.572; emphasis added). Farmers who attempt to demonstrate this cultural ideal of masculinity undermine their health – and there are many such farmers (see Courtenay, 2006).

It has been emphasised elsewhere (Rich & Stone, 1996; Courtenay & Sabo, 2001) that the negotiation of masculinity in certain contexts can present men with unique health paradoxes, particularly in regard to physical dominance and the use of violence. The perception both among some men in prison (Courtenay & Sabo, 2001) and some inner-city African American men (Rich & Stone, 1996) is that failing to fight back makes a man vulnerable to even more extreme victimisation than does retaliating. This health paradox is reflected in the 'protective, though violent, posture' described by Rich and Stone (1996, p.81): 'If you appear weak, others will try to victimise you . . . if you show yourself to be strong (by retaliating), then you are perceived as strong and you will be safe' (pp.80–81). Although these men neither actively resist nor embrace hegemonic masculinity, they are complicit in its reconstruction.

## Institutional structures, masculinities, and men's health

The institutionalised social structures that men encounter elicit different demonstrations of health-related beliefs and behaviours, and provide different opportunities to conduct this particular means of demonstrating gender. These structures – including the government and the military, corporations, the technological and healthcare industries, the judicial system, academia and the media – help to sustain gendered health risks by cultivating stereotypic forms of gender enactments and by providing different resources for demonstrating gender to women than they provide to men. Institutional structures, by and large, foster unhealthy beliefs and behaviours among men, and undermine men's attempts to adopt healthier habits (Courtenay, 2000b, 2002, 2006). The workforce is one such structure. The work that men do is the most dangerous work (see Courtenay, 2000a, 2003). Consequently, although they comprise only 56% of the US workforce, men account for nearly all (94%) fatal injuries on the job (National Institute for Occupational Safety and Health, 1993).

Although they have a profound influence on men's health, institutional structures are not simply imposed on men any more than a prescribed male sex role is simply imposed on men. 'Social structures do not exist autonomously from humans; rather . . . as we engage in social action, we simultaneously help create the social structures that facilitate/limit social practice' (Messerschmidt, 1993, p.62). Men are agents of social practice. When men demonstrate gender 'correctly', in the ways that are socially prescribed, they 'simultaneously sustain, reproduce, and render legitimate the institutional arrangements that are based on sex category' (West & Zimmerman, 1987, p.146). In a continuous cycle, definitions of gender influence social structures, which guide human interactions and social action, which in turn reinforce gendered social structures. This ongoing process results in a gender division and a differential exposure that inhibits both women and men from learning behaviours, skills and capacities considered characteristic of the 'opposite' gender (West & Zimmerman, 1987; Epstein, 1988). Men sustain and reproduce institutional structures in part for the privileges that they derive from preserving existing power structures. The businessman who works tirelessly, denies his stress, and dismisses his physical needs for sleep and a healthy diet often does so because he expects to be rewarded with money, power, position and prestige. Thus, although they are increasing their health risks, men who achieve these hegemonic ideals are compensated with social acceptance; with diminished anxiety about their manhood; and with the rewards that such normative, masculine demonstrations provide in a patriarchal society. In these regards, men also contribute to the construction of a healthcare system that ignores their gendered health concerns. Indeed, they are often the very researchers and scientists who have ignored men's gendered health risks.

## The medical institution and its constructions of gender and health

The healthcare system and its allied health fields represent a particularly important structural influence in the construction of gender and health. In the case of cardiovascular disease, for example, it is often noted that the fact that women are less likely than men to be routinely tested or treated for symptoms can foster unrealistic perceptions of risk among women

(Steingart et al., 1991; Wenger, 1994). Rarely, however, have the ways in which healthcare contributes to social constructions of men's health been examined. It has been argued that sociologists, medical researchers and other health professionals have all contributed to cultural portrayals of men as healthy and women as the 'sicker' gender (Gijsbers van Wijk et al., 1991), to strongly held beliefs that men's bodies are structurally more efficient than and superior to women's bodies (Courtenay, 2000b), and to the 'invisibility' of men's poor health status (Annandale & Clark, 1996).

As Nathanson (1977, p.148) noted over three decades ago, sex differences in health and health-related behaviour arise 'out of a medical model that has singled out women for special professional attention': 'women are encouraged and trained to define their life problems in medical terms and to seek professional help for them' (p.149). While the personal practice of participating in healthcare is constructed as feminine, the institutional practice of conducting, researching or providing healthcare is constructed as masculine and defined as a domain of masculine power. Physicians, who are primarily men, maintain power and control over the bodies of men who are not physicians and the bodies of women – as well as over male and female health professionals in lesser positions of power, such as nurses and orderlies. In these ways, the healthcare system does not simply adapt to men's 'natural' masculinity; rather, it actively constructs gendered health behaviour and negotiates among various forms of masculinity. Medical, sociological and feminist approaches to addressing gender and health have all contributed to the devaluing of women's bodies and to the privileging of men's bodies, as two feminist authors have noted (Annandale & Clark, 1996).

Historically, women but not men in the US have been encouraged to pay attention to their health (Nathanson, 1977; Lonnquist et al., 1992; Signorielli, 1993; Oakley, 1994; Annandale & Clark, 1996; Reagan, 1997). Decades of cancer education efforts in the US have been directed primarily at women (Reagan, 1997). Very rarely are educational or counselling interventions designed to reduce men's health risks (Courtenay, 2001b, 2004a, b; Stanton & Courtenay, 2003). Men also receive significantly less physician time in their health visits than women do, and generally receive fewer services and dispositions than women (see Courtenay, 2003). Men are provided with fewer and briefer explanations – both simple and technical – in medical encounters (see Courtenay, 2003). During checkups, for example, they receive less advice from physicians about changing risk factors for disease than women do. One review revealed that no study has ever found that women received less information from physicians than men, which led the authors to conclude that the findings 'may reflect sexism in medical encounters, but this may act to the advantage of female patients, who have a more informative and positive experience than is typical for male patients' (Roter & Hall, 1997, p.44).

A variety of scientific methodological factors and research methods, developed and conducted primarily by men, have also contributed to the model of deficient women's bodies (Courtenay, 2000b). For example, the use of behavioural indices of health, such as bed rest and healthcare utilisation, both pathologises women's health and underestimates men's health problems. These indices confound our understanding of morbidity, because they actually represent how men and women *cope* with illness rather than representing their true health status (Gijsbers van Wijk et al., 1991); thus they obscure what may be greater illness among men (Verbrugge, 1988; Kandrack et al., 1991). The assumption underlying these and other indices of health is that male behaviour is the normative or hidden referent; consequently, researchers and theorists alike presume that women are in poorer health because women get more bed rest than men do and see physicians more often. The terms applied to these behaviours – behaviours that can be considered health promoting – further pathologise women's health: women's *excess* bed rest and women's *over*utilisation of health services. These terms simultaneously transform curative actions into indicators of illness, make women's health problematic, and reinforce men's position in providing the standard of health or health behaviour. It has been argued that a cultural perception of men's health problems as nonexistent is required both to construct women's bodies as deficient and to reinforce women's disadvantaged social position (Annandale & Clark, 1996). To maintain this construction, 'women "cannot" be well and . . . men cannot be ill; they are "needed" to be well to construe women as sick' (Annandale & Clark, 1996, p.32). By dismissing their health needs and taking physical risks, men are legitimising themselves as the 'stronger' sex.

The poor health beliefs and behaviours that men use to demonstrate gender remain largely invisible: a testament to the potency of the social construction of men's resiliency and health. Medical and epidemiological examinations of health and health behaviour consistently fail to take into account gender, apart from biological sex. For example, while men's greater use of substances is well known, the reasons *why* men are more likely to use substances are poorly understood and rarely addressed. Similarly, although injury and death due to recreation, risk-taking and violence are always associated with being male, epidemiological and medical findings are consistently presented as if *gender* were of no particular relevance. Instead, men's risk-taking and violence are taken for granted. This failure of medical and epidemiological researchers to study and explain men's risk-taking and violence perpetuates the false, yet widespread, cultural assumption that risk-taking and violent behaviours are natural to, or inherent in, men.

## Conclusion

Research consistently demonstrates that women in the United States adopt healthier beliefs and personal health practices than men. A wealth of scientific data suggests that this distinction accounts in no small part for the fact that women suffer less severe chronic conditions and live more than five years longer than men. From a social constructionist perspective, this distinction can be understood as being among the many differences that women and men are expected to demonstrate.

If men want to demonstrate dominant ideals of manhood as defined in North American society, they must adhere to cultural definitions of masculine beliefs and behaviours and actively reject what is feminine. The resources available in the US for constructing masculinities – and the signifiers of 'true' masculinity – are largely unhealthy. Men and boys do indeed use these resources and adopt unhealthy beliefs and behaviours in order to demonstrate manhood. Although nothing strictly prohibits a man from demonstrating masculinities differently, to do so would require that he cross over socially constructed gender boundaries, and risk reproach and sometimes physical danger for failing to demonstrate gender correctly. By successfully using unhealthy beliefs and behaviours to demonstrate idealised forms of masculinity, men are able to assume positions of power, relative to women and less powerful men, in a patriarchal society that rewards this accomplishment. By dismissing their health needs and taking risks, men legitimise themselves as the 'stronger' sex. In this way, men's use of unhealthy beliefs and behaviours helps to sustain and reproduce social inequality and the social structures that, in turn, reinforce and reward men's poor health habits.

It should be noted that some men do defy social prescriptions of masculinity and adopt healthy behaviours, such as getting annual physical checkups and eating healthy foods. But although these men are constructing a form of masculinity, it is not among the dominant forms that are encouraged in men, nor is it among the forms adopted by most men. It should also be noted that women can and do adopt unhealthy beliefs and behaviours to demonstrate femininities, as in the case of unhealthy dieting to attain a culturally defined body ideal of slimness. However, as has been demonstrated elsewhere (Courtenay, 1998a, 2000b), the striving for cultural standards of femininity leads women to engage primarily in healthy, not unhealthy, behaviours.

This theory of gender and men's health will undoubtedly meet with resistance from many quarters. As a society, we all work diligently at maintaining constructions of women's health as deficient, of the female body as inferior, of men's health as ideal, and of the male body as structurally efficient and superior. From a feminist perspective, these constructions can be viewed as preserving existing power structures and the many privileges enjoyed by men in the US. Naming and confronting men's poor health status and unhealthy beliefs and behaviours may well improve their physical wellbeing, but it will necessarily undermine men's privileged position and threaten their power and authority in relation to women.

## Acknowledgement

Parts of this chapter were originally published in *Social Science & Medicine*, **50**(10).

## References

American Academy of Dermatology (1997) *"It Can't Happen to Me:" Americans Not as Safe from the Sun as They Think They Are.* Schaumburg, IL: American Academy of Dermatology.

American Cancer Society (2005) *Cancer Facts and Figures for African Americans 2005–2006.* Atlanta, GA: American Cancer Society.

American Heart Association (1995) *Heart and Stroke Facts: 1995 Statistical Supplement.* Dallas, TX: American Heart Association.

Anaya, R. (1996) "I'm the king": the macho image. In: *Muy Macho* (ed. R. Gonzales), pp.57–73. New York: Doubleday.

Annandale, E. & Clark, J. (1996) What is gender? Feminist theory and the sociology of human reproduction. *Sociology of Health and Illness*, **18**(1), 17–44.

Bohan, J.S. (1993) Regarding gender: essentialism, constructionism, and feminist psychology. *Psychology of Women Quarterly*, **17**, 5–21.

Centers for Disease Control (1995a) *Skin Cancer Prevention and Early Detection: at-a-glance.* Atlanta, GA: Centers for Disease Control.

Centers for Disease Control (1995b) Deaths from melanoma – United States, 1973–1992. *Morbidity and Mortality Weekly Report*, **44**(44), 337, 343–347.

Charmaz, K. (1995) Identity dilemmas of chronically ill men. In: *Men's Health and Illness: Gender, Power, and the Body* (eds D. Sabo & D.F. Gordon), pp.266–291. Thousand Oaks, CA: Sage Publications.

Clatterbaugh, K. (1997) *Contemporary Perspectives on Masculinity: Men, Women, and Politics in Modern Society*, 2nd edn. Boulder, CO: Westview Press.

Connell, R.W. (1992) Masculinity, violence, and war. In: *Men's Lives* (eds M.S. Kimmel & M.A. Messner), 2nd edn. pp.176–183. New York: Macmillan.

Connell, R.W. (1995) *Masculinities*. Berkeley, CA: University of California Press.

Courtenay, W.H. (1998a) Better to die than cry? A longitudinal and constructionist study of masculinity and the health risk behaviour of young American men. (University of California at Berkeley). *Dissertation Abstracts International*, **59**(08A), (Publication number 9902042).

Courtenay, W.H. (1998b) College men's health: an overview and a call to action. *Journal of American College Health*, **46**(6), 279–290.

Courtenay, W.H. (1999) *Youth* violence? Let's call it what it is. *Journal of American College Health*, **48**(3), 141–142.

Courtenay, W.H. (2000a) Behavioural factors associated with disease, injury, and death among men: evidence and implications for prevention. *Journal of Men's Studies*, **9**(1), 81–142.

Courtenay, W.H. (2000b) Engendering health: a social constructionist examination of men's health beliefs and behaviours. *Psychology of Men and Masculinity*, **1**(1), 4–15.

Courtenay, W.H. (2001a) Who are the 'men' in 'men's health?' *Society for the Psychological Study of Men and Masculinity Bulletin* (American Psychological Association), **6**(3), 10–13.

Courtenay, W.H. (2001b) Counseling men in medical settings. In: *The New Handbook of Psychotherapy and Counseling With Men: A Comprehensive Guide to Settings, Problems, and Treatment Approaches*, Vol. 1 (eds G.R. Brooks & G.E. Good), pp.59–91. San Francisco: Jossey-Bass.

Courtenay, W.H. (2002) A global perspective on the field of men's health. *International Journal of Men's Health*, **1**(1), 1–13.

Courtenay, W.H. (2003) Key determinants of the health and well-being of men and boys. *International Journal of Men's Health*, **2**(1), 1–30.

Courtenay, W.H. (2004a) Best practices for improving college men's health. In: *Developing Effective Programs and Services for College Men* (ed. G.E. Kellom), pp.59–74. San Francisco: Jossey-Bass.

Courtenay, W.H. (2004b) Making health manly: social marketing and men's health. *Journal of Men's Health and Gender*, **1**(2–3), 275–276.

Courtenay, W.H. (2006) Rural men's health: situating men's risk in the negotiation of masculinity. In: *Country Boys: Masculinity and Rural Life* (eds H. Campbell, M. Mayerfeld-Bell & M. Finney), pp.139–158. University Park, PA: Pennsylvania State University Press.

Courtenay, W.H. & Keeling, R.P. (2000a) Men, gender, and health: toward an interdisciplinary approach. *Journal of American College Health*, **48**(6), 1–4.

Courtenay, W.H. (Guest Editor) & Keeling, R.P. (2000b) Men's health: a theme issue. *Journal of American College Health*, **48**(6), 1–4.

Courtenay, W.H. & McCreary, D.R. (in press) Masculinity and gender role conflict: influence on men's likelihood of engaging in high-risk behaviors. *Sex Roles*.

Courtenay, W.H. & Sabo, D. (2001) Preventive health strategies for men in prison. In: *Confronting Prison Masculinities: The Gendered Politics of Punishment* (eds D. Sabo, T. Kupers & W. London), pp.157–172. Philadelphia, PA: Temple University Press.

Courtenay, W.H., McCreary, D.R. & Merighi, J.R. (2002) Gender and ethnic differences in health beliefs and behaviors. *Journal of Health Psychology*, **7**(3), 219–231.

Crawford, M. (1995) *Talking Difference: On Gender and Language*. Thousand Oaks, CA: Sage Publications.

Deaux, K. (1984) From individual differences to social categories: an analysis of a decade's research on gender. *American Psychologist*, **39**(2), 105–116.

Delsohn, S. (1996) *The Fire Inside: Firefighters Talk About their Lives*. New York: HarperCollins.

Department of Health and Human Services (1998) *Health, United States, 1998: Socioeconomic Status and Health Chartbook*. Hyattsville, MD: National Center for Health Statistics.

Department of Health and Human Services (2007) Deaths: Final data for 2004. *National Vital Statistics Report*, **55**(19). Hyattsville, MD: Public Health Service.

Doyal, L. (1995) *What Makes Women Sick: Gender and the Political Economy of Health*. New Brunswick, NJ: Rutgers University Press.

Eagly, A.H. (1983) Gender and social influence: a social psychological analysis. *American Psychologist*, **38**, 971–981.

Epstein, C.F. (1988) *Deceptive Distinctions: Sex, Gender, and the Social Order*. New Haven, CT: Yale University Press.

Fellows, W. (1996) *Farm Boys: Lives of Gay Men from the Rural Midwest*. Madison, WI: University of Wisconsin Press.

Geis, F.L. (1993) Self-fulfilling prophecies: a social psychological view of gender. In: *The Psychology of Gender* (eds A.E. Beall & R.J. Sternberg), pp.9–54. New York: Guilford Press.

Gerson, J.M. & Peiss, K. (1985) Boundaries, negotiation, consciousness: reconceptualising gender relations. *Social Problems*, **32**(4), 317–331.

Gibbs, J.T. (1988) Health and mental health of young black males. In: *Young, Black and Male in America: An Endangered Species* (ed. J.T. Gibbs), pp.19–257. New York: Auburn House.

Gijsbers van Wijk, C.M.T., van Vliet, K.P., Kolk, K.P. & Everaerd, W.T. (1991) Symptom sensitivity and sex differences in physical morbidity: a review of health surveys in the United States and the Netherlands. *Women and Health*, **17**, 91–124.

Goldberg, H. (1976) *The Hazards of Being Male: Surviving the Myth of Masculine Privilege*. Plainview, NY: Nash Publishing.

Golombok, S. & Fivush, R. (1994) *Gender Development*. New York: Cambridge University Press.

Hall, J.A., Roter, D.L. & Katz, N.R. (1988) Meta-analysis of correlates of provider behaviour in medical encounters. *Medical Care*, **26**, 657–675.

Harris, I., Torres, J.B. & Allender, D. (1994) The responses of African American men to dominant norms of masculinity within the United States. *Sex Roles*, **31**, 703–719.

Harrison, J. (1978) Warning: the male sex role may be dangerous to your health. *Journal of Social Issues*, **34**(1), 65–86.

Harrison, J., Chin, J. & Ficarroto, T. (1992) Warning: the male sex role may be dangerous to your health. In: *Men's Lives* (eds M.S. Kimmel & M.A. Messner), 2nd edn. pp.271–285. New York: Macmillan.

Hunter, A.G. & Davis, J.E. (1992) Constructing gender: an exploration of Afro-American men's conceptualisation of manhood. *Gender and Society*, **6**, 464–479.

Jaffe, H. (1997) Dying for dollars. *Men's Health*, **12**, 132–137, 186–187.

Kandrack, M., Grant, K.R. & Segall, A. (1991) Gender differences in health related behaviour: some unanswered questions. *Social Science and Medicine*, **32**(5), 579–590.

Kaschak, E. (1992) *Engendered Lives: A New Psychology of Women's Experience*. New York: Basic Books.

Katz, P.A. & Ksansnak, K.R. (1994) Developmental aspects of gender role flexibility and traditionality in middle childhood and adolescence. *Developmental Psychology*, **30**(2), 272–282.

Kaufman, M. (1994) Men, feminism, and men's contradictory experiences of power. In: *Theorising Masculinities* (eds H. Brod & M. Kaufman), pp.142–163. Thousand Oaks, CA: Sage Publications.

Kimmel, M.S. (1986) Introduction: toward men's studies. *American Behavioural Scientist*, **29**(5), 517–529.

Laveist, T.A. (1993) Segregation, poverty, and empowerment: health consequences for African Americans. *Milbank Quarterly*, **71**(1), 41–64.

Levant, R.F. & Majors, R.G. (1998) Masculinity ideology among African American and European American college women and men. *Journal of Gender, Culture, and Health*, **2**(1), 33–43.

Levant, R.F., Majors, R.G. & Kelley, M.L. (1998) Masculinity ideology among young African American and European American women and men in different regions of the United States. *Cultural Diversity and Ethnic Minority Psychology*, **4**(3), 227–236.

Lonnquist, L.E., Weiss, G.L. & Larsen, D.L. (1992) Health value and gender in predicting health protective behaviour. *Women and Health*, **19**(2/3), 69–85.

Majors, R. & Billson, J.M. (1992) *Cool Pose: The Dilemmas of Black Manhood in America*. New York: Touchstone.

Martin, C.L. (1995) Stereotypes about children with traditional and nontraditional gender roles. *Sex Roles*, **33**(11/12), 727–751.

Meinecke, C.E. (1981) Socialised to die younger? Hypermasculinity and men's health. *The Personnel and Guidance Journal*, **60**, 241–245.

Mermelstein, R.J. & Riesenberg, L.A. (1992) Changing knowledge and attitudes about skin cancer risk factors in adolescents. *Health Psychology*, **11**(6), 371–376.

Messerschmidt, J.W. (1993) *Masculinities and Crime: Critique and Reconceptualisation of Theory*. Lanham, MD: Rowman & Littlefield.

Messner, M.A. & Sabo, D.F. (1994) *Sex, Violence and Power in Sports: Rethinking Masculinity*. Freedom, CA: Crossing Press.

Mor, V., Masterson-Allen, S., Goldberg, R., Guadagnoli, E. & Wool, M.S. (1990) Prediagnostic symptom recognition and help seeking among cancer patients. *Journal of Community Health*, **15**(4), 253–261.

Nathanson, C. (1977) Sex roles as variables in preventive health behaviour. *Journal of Community Health*, **3**(2), 142–155.

National Institute for Occupational Safety and Health (1993) *Fatal Injuries to Workers in the United States, 1980–1989: A Decade of Surveillance* (DHHS [NIOSH] No. 93–108). Cincinnati, OH: National Institute for Occupational Safety and Health.

Oakley, A. (1994) Who cares for health? Social relations, gender, and the public health. *Journal of Epidemiology and Community Health*, **48**, 427–434.

Pappas, G., Queen, S., Hadden, W. & Fisher, G. (1993) The increasing disparity in mortality between socioeconomic groups in the United States, 1960 and 1986. *New England Journal of Medicine*, **239**(2), 103–109.

Perry, L.A., Turner, L.H. & Sterk H.M. (1992) *Constructing and Reconstructing Gender: The Links Among Communication, Language, and Gender*. Albany, NY: State University of New York Press.

Pleck, J.H. (1987) *The Myth of Masculinity*, 3rd edn. Cambridge, MA: MIT Press.

Pleck, J.H., Sonenstein, F.L. & Ku, L.C. (1994a) Problem behaviours and masculinity ideology in adolescent males. In: *Adolescent Problem Behaviours: Issues and Research* (eds R.D. Ketterlinus & M.E. Lamb), pp.165–186. Hillsdale, NJ: Lawrence Erlbaum.

Pleck, J.H., Sonenstein, F.L. & Ku, L.C. (1994b) Attitudes toward male roles among adolescent males: a discriminant validity analysis. *Sex Roles*, **30**(7/8), 481–501.

Pyke, K.D. (1996) Class-based masculinities: the interdependence of gender, class, and interpersonal power. *Gender and Society*, **10**, 527–549.

Reagan, L.J. (1997) Engendering the dread disease: women, men, and cancer. *American Journal of Public Health*, **87**(11), 1779–1787.

Rice, T.W. & Coates, D.L. (1995) Gender role attitudes in the southern United States. *Gender and Society*, **9**(6), 744–756.

Rich, J.A. & Stone, D.A. (1996) The experience of violent injury for young African-American men: the meaning of being a 'sucker'. *Journal of General Internal Medicine*, **11**, 77–82.

Roter, D.L. & Hall, J.A. (1997) *Doctors Talking with Patients/Patients Talking with Doctors: Improving Communication in Medical Visits*. Westport, CT: Auburn House.

Sabo, D. & Gordon, D.F. (1995) *Men's Health and Illness: Gender, Power and the Body*. Thousand Oaks, CA: Sage Publications.

Saltonstall, R. (1993) Healthy bodies, social bodies: men's and women's concepts and practices of health in everyday life. *Social Science and Medicine*, **36**(1), 7–14.

Signorielli, N. (1993) *Mass Media Images and Impact on Health: A Sourcebook*. Westport, CT: Greenwood Press.

Stanton, A.L. & Courtenay, W.H. (2003) Gender, stress and health. In: *Psychology Builds a Healthy World: Research and Practice Opportunities* (eds R.H. Rozensky, N.G. Johnson, C.D. Goodheart & R. Hammond), pp.105–135. Washington, DC: American Psychological Association.

Steingart, R.M., Packer, M., Hamm, P. et al. (1991) Sex differences in the management of coronary artery disease. *New England Journal of Medicine*, **325**(4), 226–230.

Street, S., Kimmel, E.B. & Kromrey, J.D. (1995) Revisiting university student gender role perceptions. *Sex Roles*, **33**(3/4), 183–201.

U.S. Preventive Services Task Force (1996) *Guide to Clinical Preventive Services*, 2nd edn. Baltimore, MD: Williams & Wilkins.

Vance, C.S. (1995) Social construction theory and sexuality. In: *Constructing Masculinity* (eds M. Berger, B. Wallis & S. Watson), pp.37–48. New York: Routledge.

Verbrugge, L.M. (1985) Gender and health: an update on hypotheses and evidence. *Journal of Health and Social Behaviour*, **26**, 156–182.

Verbrugge, L.M. (1988) Unveiling higher morbidity for men: the story. In: *Social Structures and Human Lives* (ed. M.W. Riley), pp.138–160. Thousand Oaks, CA: Sage Publications.

Verbrugge, L.M. & Wingard, D.L. (1987) Sex differentials in health and mortality. *Women and Health*, **12**(2), 103–145.

Waldron, I. (1988) Gender and health-related behaviour. In: *Health Behaviour: Emerging Research Perspectives* (ed. D. S. Gochman), pp.193–208. New York: Plenum Press.

Wenger, N.K. (1994) Coronary heart disease in women: gender differences in diagnostic evaluation. *Journal of the American Medical Women's Association*, **49**, 181–185.

West, C. & Zimmerman, D.H. (1987) Doing gender. *Gender and Society*, **1**(2), 125–151.

Williams, J.E. & Best, D.L. (1990) *Measuring Sex Stereotypes: A Multination Study*. Thousand Oaks, CA: Sage Publications.

Willits, F.K., Bealer, R.C. & Timbers, V.L. (1990) Popular images of 'rurality': data from a Pennsylvania survey. *Rural Sociology*, **55**(4), 559–578.

Woolf, S.H., Jonas, S. & Lawrence, R.S. (1996) *Health Promotion and Disease Prevention in Clinical Practice*. Baltimore, MD: Williams & Wilkins.

# Chapter 2

# POSITIONING PROSTATE CANCER AS THE PROBLEMATIC THIRD TESTICLE

John L. Oliffe

## Introduction

Writing this chapter has afforded me the opportunity to discuss what has and has *not* been said about the connections between prostate cancer and masculinities. My goal here is to provide accessible empirical, theoretical and methodological commentaries and make recommendations to engage those who have an interest in researching men's health and illness experiences using masculinity frameworks. To achieve this I have bled some 'new' data collected for my doctoral research to the existing knowledge base to illustrate, extend and perhaps challenge some of what is known, as well as predict where we might next go – both as researchers and clinicians. The chapter title is stolen, at least in part, from the wife of a prostate cancer survivor who directed the quip 'prostate cancer is our problematic third testicle' to me at a support group meeting. Her comment prompted me to think about how the prostate gland is publicly portrayed, and its estrangement from dominant discourses about men's health promotion. While these thoughts do not dominate this chapter *per se*, they do permeate as a useful backdrop to contextualise men's prostate cancer illness experiences. The final product is somewhere between pedestrian (safe!) and provocative – depending on the reader's perspective.

The statistical story of prostate cancer is typically used to describe the large numbers of men afflicted and make comparisons to other tumour sites as the interim step to arguing for dedicated research and health service resources. Indeed, the data are compelling and three epidemiological trends are particularly relevant in beginning a discussion about the connections between prostate cancer and masculinities. First, age is a known risk factor for developing prostate cancer (Albertson, 1997; Kozlowski & Grayhack, 2002). Fewer than 25% of prostate cancers occur in males younger than 65 years of age (Quinn & Babb, 2002a) and the risk of developing prostate cancer increases exponentially from 2.59% (1 in 39) in men aged between 40 and 59 years to 7.03% (1 in 14) in the 60–69 age group before doubling to 13.8% (1 in 7) among men 70 years and older (Jemal et al., 2007). The population data from industrialised nations that relates to ageing indicates that between 2007 and 2050 the percentage of persons 60 years and older will increase from 11% to 22% (United Nations, 2007). These trends are even more pronounced in countries including the United States (US) and Canada where the percentage of persons 60 years and older in 2007 is predicted to increase from 20% to 33% by 2050. One implication of living longer lives is that greater numbers of men will experience prostate cancer as a by-product of increased life expectancy.

Second, while the total number of men diagnosed with prostate cancer in western countries has steadily increased over the last 50 years, the mortality rate attributed to prostate cancer has remained constant and relatively low – especially in comparison to other cancers. For example, there were 218,890 new cases of prostate cancer in the US in 2007 and 27,090 deaths (Jemal et al., 2007). However, the vast majority of those new cases were diagnosed 'early' at either local or regional stages favouring positive prognoses (Quinn & Babb, 2002a). The net outcome of these trends is that more men are living longer with prostate cancer than ever before and, in the continued absence of a known, preventable cause or definitive cure, prostate cancer will unfold as a chronic long-term illness for many men.

Third, diverse geographic and ethnicity patterns exist for prostate cancer incidence and survival. The continent of Asia has both the lowest incidence (4.7 per 100,000 persons per year) and mortality rates (2.7 per 100,000 persons per year) in the world. The average five-year survival rate in Europe was 56% compared to 86% in the US (Quinn & Babb, 2002a). In terms of ethnicity, African Americans experience the highest rates of prostate cancer incidence and mortality worldwide, with a 47% higher incidence rate and 128% higher mortality rate than that of Caucasian men residing in the same geographic regions (Baquet et al., 1991; Boring et al., 1992; Haas et al., 1993). Immigration to western countries has revealed an increased prostate cancer incidence in Japanese men, a phenomenon linked to westernised lifestyles and changed dietary patterns (Parkin, 2001; Parkin et al., 2001). The worldwide variations in incidence and survival rates can also be attributed to different age structures in populations, disparate diagnostic technologies, variations in post-mortem cancer registrations (Quinn & Babb, 2002a, b) and the 'local' commitment to prostate cancer screening (Hsing et al., 2000). It is clear from these data that prostate cancer incidence varies considerably across the world and between ethnic groups, and it follows that men's illness experiences will also be diverse.

As illustrated by these and many other epidemiological data, prostate cancer is complex and demands sophisticated study designs and diverse research methodologies. Therefore, while biomedical researchers continue to search for the cause and cure of prostate cancer, men's illness experiences remain central to identifying and meeting the needs of those who will live and die with, as well as from, prostate cancer. Social constructionist gender frameworks, specifically the concept of plural masculinities, have been responsive to, and effective in contextualising, the aforementioned epidemiological trends. For example, masculinities researchers have focused on the identities of middle-aged and elderly men to describe their relationships to dominant ideals of masculinity in the context of living with prostate cancer. Cross-sectional studies have detailed specific points in the prostate cancer illness trajectory and often situated men's experiences in specific locales, including Canada (Gray, 2003), the United Kingdom (Chapple & Ziebland, 2002) and Australia (Broom, 2004, 2005a, b, c; Oliffe, 2004a, b, 2005, 2006a, b). So, while discrete empirical bodies of knowledge are commonly abstracted, and can appear somewhat unlinked, I suggest that masculinities research has and should continue to complement, connect and contextualise, as well as contrast the intersections of prostate cancer disease and illness. In addition, by connecting prostate cancer and masculinities, much-needed insights to middle-aged and elderly men have been derived and the challenges of living with chronic illness have been detailed to afford empirical understandings about men's experiences while detailing the diversity that can exist within *and* between men.

## A word about style

What follows is a review of the literature that explores the empirical, theoretical and methodological issues in masculinities research addressing prostate cancer. It is unpacked chronologically across the illness trajectory (i.e. from symptoms and diagnosis to the treatment[s] phase, and side effects and recovery) along with my commentary, critique and suggestions. As mentioned earlier, I have also incorporated some data drawn from my doctoral research, an ethnographic photo-elicitation study that described the experiences of 35 Anglo-Australian men who had prostate cancer. Please forgive the blending of a review with 'new' data as my somewhat ambitious intent to illustrate and extend, as well as make recommendations for advancing masculinities and prostate cancer research. In addition, my desire to share some of the PhD participant-produced photographs and revisit their narratives was fuelled by the knowledge that the poignant stories of these men might otherwise be confined to the virtual shelves that house my, and so many others', dissertations (Oliffe, 2003).

## Moving into prostate cancer

It is a useful starting point to critically consider the 'fit' between prostate cancer and dominant discourses about men's health behaviours. An emergent literature has detailed the connections between masculinities and men's health risk-taking, denial of illness and avoidance of healthcare professionals and services (Kimmel, 1994; Courtenay, 1998, 2000, 2004; Taylor et al., 1998; Watson, 2000; Lee & Owens, 2002; Robertson, 2003). However, it is important to acknowledge that in the specific context of prostate cancer some of these typical men's behaviours and their connections to masculinities are fragile at best, and perhaps redundant. For example, the cause of prostate cancer is unknown and the 'risks' for developing the disease include African American ethnicity, advanced age and family history, none of which are modifiable. Moreover, there is no definitive evidence that specific lifestyles and behaviours (including smoking tobacco, having a sedentary lifestyle, etc.) render men more susceptible to developing prostate cancer. As such, there is little evidence by which to connect men's risky behaviours and lack of self-health with the development of prostate cancer. Indeed, the inverse might be argued in many cases where prostate cancer occurs as a by-product, albeit unwanted, of living a relatively long life into the seventh, eighth or ninth decades.

Dominant forms of masculinity also idealise the male body as robust and competitive, and it often follows that health is self-assessed and affirmed by men through performance indicators such as physical and sexual prowess (Tiefer, 1987; Potts, 2000; Potts et al., 2003, 2004). When symptoms are experienced, reactive self-care is a common behaviour and typically includes medium- to long-term self-monitoring coupled with some form of self-treatment, before asking partners for advice and reluctantly seeking professional medical care (White et al., 1995; Jones, 1996; O'Hehir et al., 1997; Courtenay, 1998, 2000; Ziguras, 1998; Hayes, 2001; White, 2001; Mansfield et al., 2003). Again, some of these typical men's health behaviours hold true in prostate cancer while others are less straightforward. Many prostate cancers are present without symptoms and men often first become aware of their prostate gland when it swells up and encroaches on the urethra, hindering micturition. Early on, men often rationalise urinary changes as an artefact of older age or late-night fluid intake. The taboo nature and embarrassment of investigating urinary symptoms and/or sexual function can inhibit men from talking about, let alone *actively seeking* medical attention for urological symptoms (Pinnock et al., 1998; Chapple & Ziebland, 2002; Oliffe, 2002; Gray, 2003; Broom, 2004). Men's functional view of health is illustrated by the common scenario in which troubled 'waterworks' and multiple late-night visits to the urinal eventually lead sleep-deprived, fatigued men to seek medical advice. In terms of specific symptoms, men tend to self-triage pain as the legitimating indicator to access professional medical help. The conundrum here is that early prostate cancer is often asymptomatic, and lower urinary tract symptoms are more commonly linked to benign prostatic hypertrophy. In addition, unrelieved groin and loin pain can indicate *advanced* prostate cancer which is often accompanied by a poor prognosis. Therefore, extended self-monitoring of urinary symptoms may result in unnecessary anxiety, while waiting for specific pain sequelae can reveal a prostate cancer that is no longer amenable to curative treatments.

De-linking men's pre-existing health behaviours from prostate cancer is also reflected in the predominance of studies connecting masculinities to treatment-induced side effects of impotence and urinary incontinence. The caution here is that researchers may inadvertently represent men's prostate cancer as operating independently, without reference to established and/or shifting health and illness behaviours and beliefs. One qualitative method – life course – can provide a useful strategy to detail men's health behaviours across time and history in temporally sensitive ways (Lohan, 2007; Robertson, 2007). The approach can help to address 'context gaps' common to many cross-sectional studies (i.e. one-off, semi-structured, individual interviews) that explicitly focus on discrete moments in a cancer illness trajectory. In addition, linking health and illness behaviours inductively derives and anchors empirical accounts in what men do and do not do in specific situations, rather than assuming a 'fit' with longstanding dominant discourses about men's health behaviours.

Using a life course approach, men's behaviours and masculine identities were described across their lives in the decades leading up to prostate cancer diagnosis and following treatment (Oliffe, in press). The men's earlier health behaviours were not implicated in the development of *their* prostate cancer. Instead, the men's boyhood and middle life experiences were described to reveal the context of longstanding practices, as well as the changes that occurred over time, and in relation to prostate cancer. The study findings also detailed the intersections of structure and agency across time. For example, one participant had been a heavy smoker for much of his life. However, health promotion 'risk' messaging and linkages between tobacco and disease did not exist when he first began smoking as a young man during the 1940s and 1950s. The study participants also explained that when they were ill, treatment(s) through public hospital-based services, rather than self-health and illness prevention, prevailed as the socially affirmed and government supported way to treat disease up until the 1970s. These and other important details afforded by life course methods provided insights to the men's behaviours, and direction for the design and implementation of interventions targeted to supporting prostate cancer survivors of similar demographics and age.

Men's poor health outcomes have also been linked to professional health services, and numerous studies have highlighted the challenges when men access medical services. For example, men and their enactments of masculinity can be puzzling for medical professionals (Moynihan, 1998; Banks, 2001; Seymour-Smith et al., 2002) and men's experiences of healthcare institutions and interactions with professionals can dissuade them from accessing services (Courtenay, 2000). Men's avoidance of health services has been linked to 'male unfriendly' waiting rooms (Heesacker et al., 1999), healthcare professionals' preoccupation with changing men's behaviours (Watson, 2000) as well as the anonymity, marginalisation and subordination that can occur when men enter healthcare institutions (Courtenay, 2000). When men engage professional help they commonly experience difficulty expressing their concerns (Courtenay, 2000) and present in clinical practice as hypo-emotional (Honkalampi et al., 1999) or alexithymic (Grossman & Wood, 1993; Wilhelm et al., 2002) and forget (Aneshensel et al., 1987), fail to report (Pescorosolido & Boyer, 1999; Angst et al., 2002) or minimise or trivialise their symptoms (O'Brien et al., 2005).

## Approaching diagnosis

Understanding the intersections between men's behaviours and health services are especially relevant to prostate cancer for two reasons. First, the digital rectal examination (DRE), which includes the insertion of a lubricated gloved finger to the rectum to palpate the prostate gland through the rectal wall, has historically been the primary diagnostic test and is poorly tolerated by men (Macias et al., 2000; Nagler et al., 2005), particularly those of lower socioeconomic status (Dale et al., 1999) and African American ethnicity (Forrester-Anderson, 2005). In the late 1980s, the prostate-specific antigen (PSA) blood test became available and, although governments and cancer councils have never recommended prostate cancer screening in western countries, there is strong evidence that the rates of de facto screening in men over 50 years old, and especially those aged between 60 and 69 years, are remarkably high (Smith et al., 1998).

Although it is recommended that general practitioners (GPs) and patients discuss screening information prior to testing, including the implications of an abnormal result, there is little scientific evidence on which to advise patients about the benefits of prostate cancer screening (Chan & Sulmay, 1998; Pinnock et al., 1998; Ward et al., 1998; Dunn & Kirk, 2000; Cancer Council Australia, 2007).

Second, there are divergent medical opinions about whether detection of prostate cancer will result in benefits for patients (Cancer Council Australia, 2007) because cancers of the prostate do not act predictably and vary from those that are indolent, slow-growing tumours that cause few changes to men's lives, to those that are aggressive and lethal. When diagnosed, the decision whether to treat intermediate tumours is particularly challenging because there is no precise way to predict which tumours in this group will be non-threatening or lethal (Laws et al., 2000). The perception of prostate cancer as an older man's disease that men die *with*, rather than *of* (Albertson, 1997; Gorman, 2002) is also supported by much of the epidemiological data. This makes it arduous to estimate the 'value', in terms of extra years of life versus quality of life afforded by prostate cancer detection through screening and subsequent treatment(s).

It is fair to say that the lack of scientific evidence about the virtues of screening and/or treating prostate cancer might influence and legitimise some men's avoidance of doctors. The ideals of informed consent and patient autonomy can be disrupted by biomedical cultures that routinely screen, diagnose and treat cancers, often in quick succession. For example, an abnormal PSA result can mark the beginning of a slippery slope in which men find themselves with little time or opportunity to fully consider their options or the potential impact of treatments (Oliffe, 2006a). Prostate cancer screening is distinct and somewhat estranged from other health promotion screens such as cholesterol checks. However, ironically, cholesterol and PSA can be 'bundled', requiring a single serum sample, and included in routine checkups by some physicians. Men who default PSA screening decisions to their GP without understanding the implications of an abnormal result are reliant on the GP's beliefs and perceptions of due diligence rather than acting on their own health beliefs.

In the last few years, the PSA velocity (doubling time of the PSA value) rather than a single PSA score has been used increasingly by some prostate cancer specialists to gauge the need for a definitive diagnosis and/or treatment. One emergent change to the clinical management of prostate cancer, referred to as active surveillance (regularly monitoring PSA and biopsy values without actively treating low-grade prostate cancers) suggests that *some* men will have the option of delaying treatment (Pickles et al., 2007). This might positively influence men to access healthcare professionals for prostate cancer screening; however, it may also affirm many men's perceptions that there is little need to know (and therefore worry) about the existence of a cancer that does not need immediate treatment (Oliffe et al., in press).

The majority of men who have an abnormal PSA and/or DRE screen or test will require a transrectal ultrasound biopsy (TRUS-Bx) as a means to definitively diagnose prostate cancer (Laws et al., 2000). The TRUS-Bx involves the passing of biopsy needles through the rectal wall to the prostate gland. Tiny pieces of tissue, typically between 6 and 12 samples, are removed from the prostate via the needles. The TRUS-Bx is invasive and has potential side effects including haemorrhage, systemic infection (septicaemia), psychological stress (Taylor, 1993; Hirst et al., 1996; Chan & Sulmay, 1998), anxiety, pain and occasionally impotence (Zisman et al., 1999, 2001; Kim, 2000; Oliffe, 2004a, b; Chapple et al., 2007). The psychological stressors and pain experienced by men during TRUS-Bx has attracted some research attention, and these issues featured prominently in my interviews with Australian men.

**Scenario 1:** The penetration and pain of transrectal ultrasound biopsy

During my doctoral fieldwork I was surprised to learn that in Australia the TRUS-Bx was often administered without local or systemic analgesia. Many men described significant pain, and one participant (T.C.) shared photograph 1 and a narrative that highlighted the context, as well as the specificities, of his TRUS-Bx. He began his account by recalling the halcyon days of 1994:

*I'd just come back from a trip overseas. I had money in the bank. I had a good business. I had a future ahead of me. I was going to work until I dropped. I was never going to retire, blah, blah, blah, I was King Dick.*

All that changed when T.C., at 54 years of age, woke up one morning in 1996 and was unable to move. An X-ray revealed a fractured vertebra which left him lying flat on his back for the remainder of the year. In 1998 he was granted a disability pension, but by that stage his one-man subcontracting business had disappeared. During this two-year period his brother was diagnosed with prostate cancer and his mother-in-law died of lung cancer. In addition, T.C. was increasingly getting up during the night to pass urine. Yet, it was knee pain and the need for an analgesic prescription that eventually prompted him to see a GP. During the consultation, the GP performed a routine

DRE which revealed an enlarged prostate, a finding that prompted T.C. to tell the doctor 'My father had benign prostate hyper-trophy . . . my brother is in remission for prostate cancer and I am going to the toilet six times a night.' A TRUS-Bx followed shortly thereafter and T.C. pointed to a bike pump (see photograph) in sum-marising his experience of that procedure:

> *You have a bloody great rod jammed up your anus . . . the insertion was bad enough but the worst part is that you could feel it flicking around deep inside you . . . probing.*

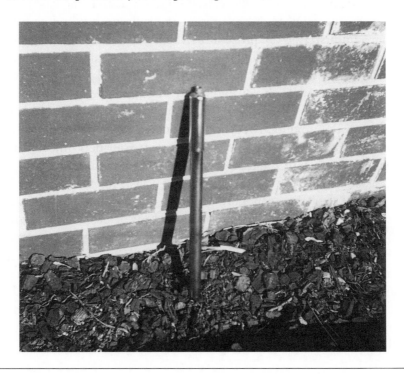

T.C.'s photograph and narrative help us to understand what underpinned his anxiety, discomfort and subsequent protest about the TRUS-Bx. It was clear that his linkages to dominant ideals of masculinity had been eroded over time, initially as a consequence of injury and then illness, which in turn affected his ability to work and maintain his lifestyle, let alone accu-mulate wealth. Moreover, as these significant life changes unfolded, T.C. was exposed to the cancer and illness experiences of others. As evidence of *his* cancer accrued, the TRUS-Bx results threatened to take him even further away from the masculine ideals he had embodied and enjoyed.

Disdain for the means by which the diagnosis was reached focused on the physicality of being penetrated anally during the TRUS-Bx, as is clearly represented by the bike pump in the photograph and the accompanying narrative. Although penetration is one of many issues at play here, it provides a legitimate 'place' to protest the means and manner by which his prostate cancer was diagnosed. In summating the experience, T.C. quipped 'a more graphic description of what was going to happen (during the TRUS-Bx) might have helped . . . but, then again, probably if I had known that, it would have made me even more worried'.

Another significant TRUS-Bx related finding was that the vast majority of the men I interviewed did not report their discomfort and pain to the clinician administering the procedure. It is likely that men's longstanding stoicism and alliance to 'toughing it out' had informed, at least in part, the continued practice of not providing TRUS-Bx analgesia in many Australian clinics. As such, men's endurance of pain helped to minimise the time, cost and 'fuss' in getting the diagnostic job done. In an attempt to follow up on this finding, I recently conducted field work in a Canadian hospital and found that local anaesthetic was routinely injected to the margins of the prostate gland prior to the TRUS-Bx procedure. One of the clinicians administering the TRUS-Bx was a visiting physician who was quick to point out (while conducting a TRUS-Bx procedure) that Australian men must be much tougher because he had never *needed* to administer TRUS-Bx analgesia in Australia. This scenario illustrates how masculinities are performance based, guided and governed by cultural ideals about how men should be, and actively constructed within hierarchies. The connections between TRUS-Bx and masculinities are further discussed elsewhere (Broom, 2004; Oliffe, 2004a, b; Chapple et al., 2007), and it is clear that many men experience enormous challenges in the moments and months of moving into a diagnosis of prostate cancer.

## Moving through prostate cancer

A diagnosis of prostate cancer places most men promptly under the care of a prostate cancer specialist (e.g. urologist or radiation oncologist). This can challenge both patient and physician, as they try to address complex cancer-related issues without the benefits of having an established relationship. The patient–physician relationship is also likely to be ongoing and long term, a situation that repeatedly contravenes dominant ideals about men's self-reliance and avoidance of healthcare professionals and medical services. A secondary analysis of interview data drawn from Australian and Canadian men revealed particular features of patient–physician prostate cancer communication in the male dyad (Oliffe & Thorne, 2007). For example, hierarchical power relationships played out in patient–physician interactions, with some men conceding authority, knowledge and access to physicians, and others reporting a reduction of anxiety when the physician's use of humour or affability reduced that power imbalance. Protest masculinities were also evident when men interpreted the delivery and/or content of what physicians said as overtly subordinating. Broom's (2005a, b, c) work solicited the views of prostate cancer specialists as well as patients to contextualise how masculinities can be negotiated in ways that rely on, or alternatively minimise, power relations. Broom (2005c) found that accessing prostate cancer information and/or support online enabled some patients to take control and limit their inhibitions in face-to-face encounters with physicians. He also suggested that online forums could provide the anonymity for men to manage the constraints posed by dominant constructions of masculinity, but warned that some prostate cancer specialists perceived online resources as a threat to their expert status (Broom, 2005b). Drawing on the same data set Broom (2005a) clarified that many prostate cancer specialists also acknowledged that web-based information could contribute positively to their relationships with patients.

There is a significant need to further develop understandings about what and where patients access materials, and how they use that information to self-manage and engage with healthcare professionals and services. Following the lead of Broom (2005a, b, c) it is vital to also make available opportunities for healthcare professionals to discuss their experiences of treating men for prostate cancer. By talking about men and masculinity, healthcare professionals can formally consider and articulate their ideas about what underpins men's health behaviours, and their perceptions of 'good' and 'bad' cancer communication and therapeutic relations. This 'both sides of the story' approach offers important insights to develop and mobilise strategies that are mindful of how structures (hospitals, policies and funding) can influence healthcare professionals' delivery of services. In addition, the collection of patient–physician dyad data can afford comparisons to detail the many complex connections between structure and agency as the foundation to prescribing feasible interventions and future healthcare services.

It is in the aftermath of a prostate cancer diagnosis and treatment(s) that the vast majority of masculinities research can be found. Treatment side effects, especially impotence, have been the focus of numerous studies dedicated to describing men's masculine identities in relation to hegemonic ideals. Fergus and colleagues (2002) were among the first to connect masculinities and prostate cancer in a grounded theory study of 18 men who had experienced sexual dysfunction following various treatments. They described the core category 'preservation of manhood', which detailed men's sexual behaviours and beliefs across the trajectory including:

(a) attempts to increase the chances of survival while endeavouring to minimise the extent of sexual impairment;
(b) the perception of sexual dysfunction as disrupting gender identity;
(c) stigmatisation regarding diminished sexual capabilities;
(d) self-imposed pressure to continue providing and deriving sexual satisfaction;
(e) active efforts to minimise, contain or overcome the loss.

Although the study participants attempted to work around the loss – and some eventually achieved acceptance – few participants were able to deny the magnitude of the losses as a result of sexual dysfunction. A narrative analysis of 3 of these 18 study participants provided further insights about how each man renegotiated performances of masculinity, the majority of which occurred within the parameters of performance consistent with hegemonic masculinity (Gray et al., 2002). The study findings revealed that impotence can be a big deal for some men, and is at least a concern for most. However, the authors warned against making assumptions about fixed relationships between men's sexual practices and masculinity.

Studies by Arrington (2003), Broom (2004) and Oliffe (2005) highlighted similar impotence-related issues and there is strong agreement that initially, for most men, the risk of death greatly outweighs the prospects of living with erectile dysfunction (ED). Most men prioritise treatment and risk ED as a means to living longer. This objective, rational choice can shift in the post-treatment period and many men attempt to regain their erectile function. Across studies, the means to achieving this were not without internal and external tensions. For example, some elderly men grappled with dominant ideals that 'old' men did not need sex or should not be interested in having sex because it did not accurately reflect their sexualities and desires (Arrington, 2003). Although there is also much marketing of ED treatments, many men were uncertain about the appropriateness of using products and prostheses to achieve an erection. It is here, in the ambiguities, contradictions and tensions that most masculinities studies have revealed important details about how men reformulate and/or rely on dominant ideals about erection, penetration and climax models of male sex.

**Scenario 2:** The visible anonymity of treating erectile dysfunction

An example of the tensions that can underpin ED and its treatments was evident in the way Arthur, a 46-year-old post-prostatectomy patient, defended his reliance on a penetrative model of sex, yet simultaneously felt conspicuous by the visibility of needing help to achieve that ideal. During our interview, Arthur pointed to the photograph included here and explained that the urologist had given him 'this totally anonymous, completely unsexy brown paper bag'. Initially it contained absorbent pads for urinary incontinence, then a vacuum erection device (VED) to treat his ED. Arthur suggested the bag implied 'this problem [ED] is to be hushed up', yet rather than providing anonymity, it actually identified him:

*Like policemen in plain clothes stand out . . . it's like here's a brown paper bag. 'You can't get it up' that's what this bag says to you and as you walk out through the waiting room there are half a dozen other men . . . sometimes with their partners or younger children and they all look at you and see you walk out with a brown paper bag and even though it is meant to be anonymous it is . . . definitely a sign you are in the club.*

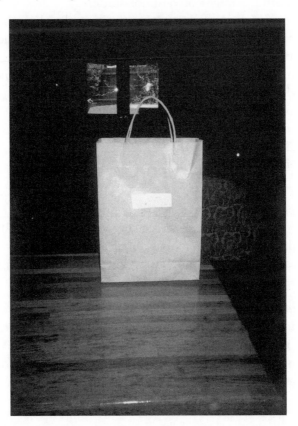

Arthur's photograph and story illustrated the plurality of masculinities in the way he wanted to treat his ED, but did not want to be identified as impotent by others, or seen as needing help to achieve a full (i.e. potent) recovery following surgery. As a relatively young man (in comparison to the typical prostate cancer population) he situated himself as distinctly different, biologically needing to re-establish his potency to enact the desires of an 'intact' middle-age libido. In what followed in our interview, Arthur described in detail his experiences of numerous ED treatments and, despite his limited success, he shared his future hopes and plans for re-instating potency. In terms of analyses, I suggested that he was reliant on dominant ideals of masculinity that prescribe erection, penetration and climax as men's sexuality (Oliffe, 2005). That said, his, and many other men's narratives indicated expectations for recapturing previous sexual function rather than rehabilitating to an altered functionality. Perceptions of having failed scientifically proven ED treatments occurred for many men, and the lack of spontaneity in having to schedule sex and changes to how sex 'felt' also resulted in most men reformulating masculine ideals to take up more feminine ways, including touching and petting, to express their love. While most studies indicate that men try to address their ED through various means but eventually resolve to live with their ED, this 'position' is neither straightforward nor static.

Although the functional aspects of men's sexuality have been linked to masculinities, treatment-induced changes to the body aesthetics, specifically reductions in penis and testes size and the development of breasts (i.e. gynaecomastia) have attracted less attention. The details about these changes provide intriguing and complex terrain in which to consider the conditions under which men's bodies operate (Oliffe, 2005, 2006b).

**Scenario 3:** The size aesthetic

I was struck by the openness of a corporate lawyer, Patrick, who had his wife, Victoria, take a series of seven photographs, all of which were similar to the one included here and featured his penis and surgical scar following prostatectomy. During our interview, Patrick explained:

*There are two reasons for having those photos, one is to show the scar which effectively runs from the navel right down to as far as you can go without doing some other damage. And the other one is . . . to show that the penis, I believe, is shorter than it was.*

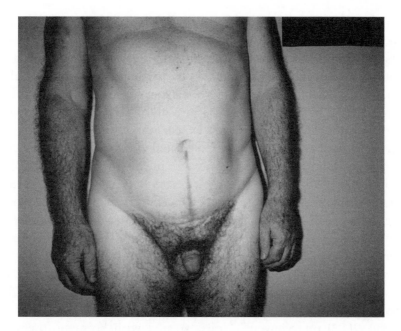

Patrick explained that in the course of taking out the prostate gland the surgeon had to cut off the urethra just where it entered the bladder, and that pulled it up and appeared to shorten his penis. Patrick 'wasn't aware of that [penis shortening] in advance' of the surgery and 'asked the urologist about it . . . he said "yes it sometimes happens like that"'. Patrick did not 'have any problem about that':

> It is no real concern. It is just the way it is. I am told if and when it does become erect it would be the same size as it would have been anyway so that doesn't, that is not an issue.

It is important to note that disuse atrophy is often the core problem in penile shortening, a detail that Patrick was unaware of. During our interview Patrick spoke objectively about the physical changes and reconciled the unexpected damage because being alive was the most important thing. Unlike other surgeries, aesthetic changes to external genitalia were not necessarily anticipated because the prostate gland resides inside the body and is not directly linked to the penis. The penis biologically and socially differentiates men from women (Martino & Pallotta-Chiarolli, 2003) and size can inform masculine hierarchies in which the large penis is socially constructed as superior and more likely to deliver the promise of sexual prowess (Edgar, 1997). Therefore, men may be emasculated by reduced penis size as well as ED. However, the lack of information about the possibility of aesthetic as well as functional changes prior to treatments is perhaps the most significant issue here. The taken-for-granted acceptance and explanations extracted by participants from medical staff illustrates the power, contradictions and expectations of men's bodies, and the pressures to be a 'sturdy oak' despite unforeseen losses in pursuing a longer life through treating prostate cancer.

Advanced prostate cancers are often treated with hormone therapies that block the production of testosterone as a means to slowing the cancer's spread to other parts of the body. A few researchers have focused on various hormone therapies in outlining the changes to men's bodies. Navon and Morag (2003a, b, 2004) published three articles from a qualitative interview study of 15 men who received hormone therapy. One thematic finding, 'maleness without a full sense of masculinity' described how body feminisation following hormone therapy resulted in a 'betwixt and between state' in which participants did not feel fully male nor did they define themselves as feminine (Navon & Morag, 2004, p.2341). Chapple and Ziebland (2002) interviewed 32 men treated with hormone therapy for prostate cancer about the effects on their masculinity, and revealed profound effects on libido, energy, ability to work, body shape and competitiveness. In a study of 15 men treated with hormones I found similar issues (Oliffe, 2006b) and one participant in particular, 'Randwick', provided fascinating insights to the body changes he experienced.

**Scenario 4:** The body unknown

Randwick began talking about the photograph included here (which has been cropped to protect his identity) by quipping that he had 'breasts . . . I [he] think some of the females would be quite happy to have'. However, as our discussion continued he revealed a great deal about the complexities and contradictions of living in a body that he perceived as not male:

> From the neck down to the waist, it's not my normal body. I've always had a truck driver's body, because I've always been a working person . . . now, that body to me is not mine.

Randwick told the story of his body over time; he described a muscular working-class body from the past and asserted 'there are truck drivers and then there are truck drivers'. He explained that he was a real truck driver because he not only drove the truck, he packed and

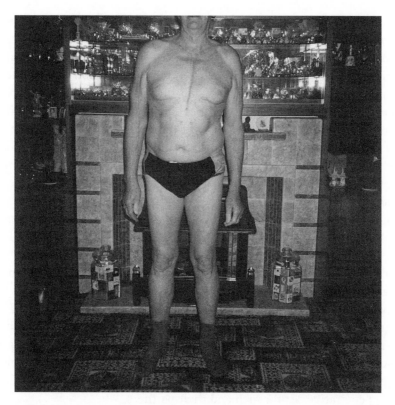

unpacked the load that it carried. This demanded strength and muscularity which his normal masculine body provided. However, the body in the photograph had been invaded by an unfamiliar feminine torso. Breasts disrupted Randwick's perceptions of how his masculine body should look, as it was not a 'true' representation of his body, its history or its achievements. His working-class body was missing, yet Randwick was surrounded by working-class achievements. Indeed, the entire backdrop in this photograph is filled with trophies from, and signifiers of, a successful marriage and working-class life. Yet, the body at the forefront betrays those achievements. Randwick, at 74 years of age, revealed how muscle and tone can be enduring aspirations and signifiers of masculinity regardless of age. Indeed, the masculine body was so important to Randwick that he no longer swam without a shirt for fear that he would be seen by others as having breasts, and therefore, suspect, and only 'part' man. Being complicit in sustaining masculine ideals about how men's bodies look and operate informed his strategy to conceal his 'abnormalities'.

Prostate cancer hormone therapies have also provided fertile ground to further theorise the intersections of gender and sex. Based on their study, Chapple and Ziebland (2002) concluded that gender is largely a social construction, but hormones, and therefore essentialism, subtly affect the way men and women react to each other and how gendered roles are embodied. Further, they recommended that, rather than duality, 'the physical body as well as culture should be considered when trying to explain what it means to be masculine, and how illness may affect men's sense of masculinity' (Chapple & Ziebland, 2002, p.820). Wassersug has taken a pragmatic approach in arguing against the marginality associated with, and the derogatory use of, the term 'eunuch' that can be used to label men who are treated with hormone therapies (Gray et al., 2005; Aucoin & Wassersug, 2006). He also proposes a gender variant outside the man-woman duality (Wassersug & Johnson, 2007). Eloquently, he mobilises these perspectives to disrupt biomedical ideals about treating ED by detailing non-coital alternatives (including dildos and sex toys) and highlighting *all* the possibilities for men's sex and sexualities (Gray & Klotz, 2004; Warkentin et al., 2006; Wasserug & Oliffe, in press). This is important work because as a prostate cancer survivor, and biologist and sociologist, Wassersug has integrated sex (the biology of testosterone) and gender (the social construction of masculinities) analyses in theoretically innovate ways but, perhaps more importantly, he offers empirically supported alternatives to penetrative sex for men and their partners.

## Moving out from prostate cancer

More than a decade ago Charmaz (1995) suggested 'time distance' from diagnosis and treatment was an important predictor of the level of men's grief and loss and detailed the public and private representations that men embodied in the context of living with chronic illness. Similarly, prostate cancer 'recovery' stories can provide important insights about how men move out and away from illness cultures. Men's stoicism about health and illness matters has been described over many years, and no doubt many men ascribe to silence rather than the self-disclosure explored by Wassersug (in press) regarding *their* prostate cancer. However, increasingly visible are masculine templates that have emerged to show how men can speak publicly about prostate cancer, as evidenced by the testimonials of well-known men including Arnold Palmer, Charlton Heston, Colin Powell, Robert De Niro, Sean Connery, Rudy Giuliani, Bob Dole, Sidney Poitier, Harry Belafonte and General Norman Schwarzkopf. The power of celebrity has afforded men legitimacy in acknowledging and courageously moving through their prostate cancer with varying degrees of self-disclosure. These stories consistently position men's self-disclosure as the lynchpin for raising both public awareness and research dollars to identify the cause and/or cure for prostate cancer. The good fight and traditional masculine ideals embodied and endorsed by celebrities can also offer important direction and hope for other men. I have observed instances when 'ordinary' men use prostate cancer support groups as a platform to embody similar practices, using dynamism language and masculine metaphors to detail their prostate cancer fight (Oliffe et al., 2008; Bottorff et al., 2008). These examples of men's talk are encouraging. However, many men cannot and will not discuss their prostate cancer experiences publicly, and for these men moving out from prostate cancer is often tentative and conditional, demanding both stoicism and self-disclosure, depending on where and whom they are with.

**Scenario 5:** Almost hegemonic

I doubt I will ever forget the first interview with Ben, a 51-year-old engineer with a PhD who had recently undergone a prostatectomy. He was visibly distressed and consumed by the impotence and urinary incontinence that he unexpectedly endured following treatment. The interview meandered across an entire afternoon, punctuated only by a brief coffee break in which the tape recorder was turned off but the dialogue continued, refocusing on Ben's prostate cancer. His narratives were steeped in anxiety, fear and palpable decisional regret in having chosen surgery as the most effective means to ridding himself of an early-stage cancer. He explained an internal conflict in that he harboured two discordant, conflicted personas, the visibility of which depended on where he was and who he was with. He explained these issues through the photograph shown below.

*This is to represent the fact there's a real me and there's an image of me ... I give out two stories ... there's a degree of false-ness ... For most people, certainly at work ... 'How are you [Ben]?' 'I'm great. Fine'. 'How was the operation?' 'Really good.' 'What was the outcome?' 'Excellent.' ... Now that is story number 1, but story number 2 ... there is incontinence ... far worse than I expected ... I didn't understand it would be like that ... I'm extremely disappointed ... and the impotence is worse than I expected, and they are not trivial matters. They are not going away. They are permanent life-long problems. They are irreversible. So, there are two really different stories here.*

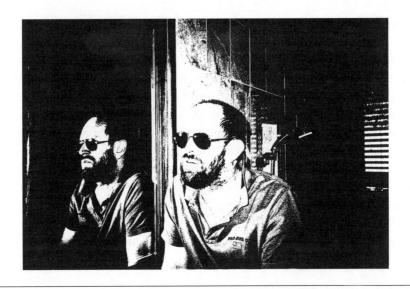

The photograph captures Ben and his reflection to represent his assured public hegemonic masculine self which is preserved at work by assuring colleagues that all is well. His private identity is one of disablement and marginalisation, uncertain about his ability to cope with the unexpected morbidities. The reflection and the real, the public and private, the hegemonic and marginalised co-exist in perpetual awkwardness and conflict. Ben is powerful yet powerless, in control yet out of control, wealthy yet poor. He suggested that in not speaking up about his dissatisfaction and poor outcomes, 'the public probably sees . . . no problems with this health system', and he wanted other 'men to have better choices'. However, 'there is a privacy issue, and also I don't want to be a perpetual moaner'.

I returned to interview Ben again some four months later, and was struck by the contrast. With a spry affect and an air of optimism he greeted me enthusiastically. I was relieved and eager to talk, hopeful, as if Ben was about to tell me that he was continent and potent. Instead he told me he had been promoted by his employer and was moving interstate. We talked about the concept of 'ceilings' in organisations, where employees often reach their potential as judged by management at one organisation and have to move to another for promotion. Ben smiled and suggested:

*I [he] might have just reached it [the ceiling], but it wasn't where I'd been sitting for the last ten years . . . there's still plenty of exciting things to do, so I won't be worrying about 'ceilings' for a little while.*

Ben's masculine identity closely aligned to work and career, and a promotion, interstate move and the supervision of new staff provided him with the opportunity to focus on what was working in an effort to resolve his internal disputation. The job promotion provided a safe, valued place to move out from illness cultures by confirming Ben's expertise and ability to successfully compete, in ways that overshadowed and downplayed his prostate cancer and treatment-induced morbidities. As our interview came to an end it was obvious that Ben's disclosure about his prostate cancer was complete; he had returned to work.

## Conclusion

The social construction of masculinities has provided the epistemological and ontological freedoms to explore and contextualise men's prostate cancer illness experiences. The plurality of masculinities (Connell, 1995) has afforded nuanced accounts to confirm, as well as contradict, what is often espoused as cutting across all men's health and illness issues. This is important because the interconnectedness of gender, culture and social class that influence men's diverse and shifting health behaviours (as contrasted to the uniform and unchangeable behaviours attributed to essentialised testosterone-driven maleness) offers something for policy-makers, clinicians and researchers to work with, rather than to change (Oliffe & Bottorff, 2006). The concept of hegemonic masculinity that details cultural ideals about men's power (in relation to women as well as other men) and masculine characteristics (e.g. self-reliance, stoicism, sexual prowess) has also been used to describe and contrast what men do (and do not do) when confronted by and living with prostate cancer. This work has provided an important foundation.

However, perhaps inevitably, the limits of description and diversity have begun to emerge, and the need to theoretically advance analyses to produce interventions rather than rerun the well-established connections between prostate cancer and masculinities have become an integral follow-up. This imperative is, in large part, dictated by individuals and collectives that fund research and their obligations to those who provide and consume prostate cancer care. Specifically, issues of prostate cancer are increasingly linked to service provision and the political and financial pressures, along with public expectations about access to effective healthcare, inform distinct demands. As such, many 'health' services in their current 'leaner and meaner' incarnations are hungry for more than sociological theorising about the connections between prostate cancer and masculinities.

Policy-makers, clinicians and health researchers alike crave 'something' more than descriptions and theory to hang their expert and interventionist hats upon. Said another way, *if we accept that masculinities and prostate cancer are inextricably linked, what is it that we can do with that knowledge to improve men's lives and clinical services?* After all, men's diversity might offer little practical help for clinicians who want to anticipate, interpret and effectively deal with behaviours common to men who arrive in their clinical practice. The measurement of masculinity, although epistemologically at odds with social constructions of masculinity, offers the utopia, at least for some, of 'nailing down' masculinity so that it can be generalised and accounted for (Addis & Mahalik, 2003; Mahalik et al., 2003). This seems reasonable because descriptive accounts about men's diversity, in and of themselves, do not map clinical pathways for prostate cancer. *Or do they?*

I acknowledge that the first step to providing a solution is to describe the problem, and this has, at least in part, been addressed by the published, empirically based articles that link prostate cancer and masculinities. By talking with men about their prostate cancer, important understandings and insights have been developed. To build on this foundation, three incremental steps are necessary.

First, the surfacing dissatisfaction about the limits of relying on diversity to account for men's varied alignments to masculine ideals requires thoughtful consideration. It is important to note that many study participants represented in the prostate cancer and masculinities research have been recruited through support groups, and it could be argued that what *we* have collectively described is largely an artefact of the prostate cancer support group phenomenon. This is limiting because such support groups attract western, white middle-class, educated men. Clearly, this is a narrow definition of diversity that significantly limits the representativeness and usability of those study findings when considering the needs of other groups of men who are affected by prostate cancer. Similarly, it is important to note that most empirical accounts detail the experiences of war baby and baby boomer generations, and these findings are limited in what they can say about or predict for future generations of prostate cancer survivors. Therefore, I suggest that the current lack of diversity limits description in ways that can inhibit the translation of those findings to interventions. From a theoretical perspective, hegemonic masculinity is also implicated in its current myopic representation of diversity. Galdas et al. (2005) pointed out that hegemonic masculinity is consistently western and white-centric. Taking this a step further, I suggest that hegemonic masculinity is the dead man walking in men's health research; and proliferation – the plurality of hegemonic masculinities – might best achieve a stay of execution. Said another way, it is time to explicitly ask study participants about *their* masculine ideals to anchor specific hegemonic masculinities in men's lives as well as to contextually describe individual patterns of association.

Second, there is a need to know more about gender relations and how they connect to men's experiences of prostate cancer. This can best be achieved by talking with the partners of men and/or conducting interviews among couple-dyads to better understand how gender relations are negotiated and performed in the context of prostate cancer. Similarly, more information is required about the gendered expectations and performances of healthcare providers, and the gender ideals represented and embodied in healthcare institutions. Such information will assist with 'teasing out' how masculine identities are negotiated and the influence of femininities on men's prostate cancer-related behaviours and beliefs.

Third, teaching gender to healthcare professionals (both students and practicing clinicians) needs to include masculinities. Gender and health have related predominantly to women's health issues. In marketing terms, the connections between masculinities and men's health and illness issues such as prostate cancer need to be made visible and embedded within health curricula, rather than an 'add on' or competitor to women's health or breast cancer. Achieving this is important to legitimising gender as a determinant of health (Frank et al., 2007), and pivotal to soliciting the support of politicians, policy-makers and clinicians to ultimately benefit all cancer 'patients'.

In closing, I want to explain why I have called this chapter *Positioning Prostate Cancer as the Problematic Third Testicle*. I have often wondered what it would take to highlight the qualities of the gland as a means to promote pampering of the prostate. A 'makeover' might reposition the gland as worthy of targeted health promotion programmes, rather than continuating to rely on pathology and risk. For example, in terms of anatomy and physiology, the prostate gland is, arguably, the king of male glands. The muscular walnut-sized gland is unique to the male body, a masterpiece of engineering design marking the nexus of men's urinary, sexual and reproductive systems. Microscopically, fluids and secretions in their own liquefied natures move in ways that defy gravity (Vilas, 2003). The gland produces most of the semen, the milky fluid transporting the sperm, and contributes 70% of the total volume of men's ejaculate. Less often discussed are the linkages between the prostate gland and men's sexualities. Queer theory has been most forthright in acknowledging the prostate as a site of pleasure and detailing how massage can heighten arousal, explicitly attributing the pulsating pleasures of the male orgasm to the glands' contractility during ejaculation. Yet, despite the inherent maleness of the prostate and its unencumbered linkages to men's reproductive health it has remained somewhat muted, subordinate to other biological markers such as the penis and testes. This is, in part, related to the positioning of the gland inside the body, as well as the brooding pathology that may or may not reveal itself in men's middle or later years. So, in closing, I propose that the prostate gland be reconceptualised as much more than a potential site of trouble. Rather, the prostate should be recognised as a site of anatomical wonder, worthy of self-awareness and health, and 'good' publicity rather than the 'time bomb' scenario so commonly put forward to crudely encourage its surveillance and dismantling. Of course, the specificities of how this might be achieved will feature elsewhere, hopefully in the near future.

## Author note

The data used for this section is drawn from my PhD, an ethnographic photo-elicitation study of 35 Anglo-Australian heterosexual men who had prostate cancer. The data collected for that study has provided empirical, theoretical and methodological insights that are published elsewhere (Oliffe 2004b, 2005, 2006a, b; Oliffe & Bottorff, 2006; Oliffe & Thorne, 2007; Oliffe, in press). This chapter borrows from some of those works, but seeks to extend the analysis by focusing on the body, the prostate gland and its connections to masculinities.

## Acknowledgements

Sincere thanks to the men whose stories and photographs were pivotal to my doctoral studies. You have enabled me to share your insights in an effort to help others. It is with mixed emotions that I have penned our final telling in this chapter. Hopefully, the narratives and images will live on to inform and inspire, as well as bear testimony to the value of speaking up and out. The writing of this chapter was made possible by the generous career support provided by a Canadian Institutes of Health Research (Institute of Gender and Health) New Investigator award and a Michael Smith Foundation for Health Research Scholar award. Thanks also to Richard Wassersug, Melanie Phillips, Andrea Becking and Tina Thornton for their thoughtful reviews of earlier drafts of this chapter.

# References

Addis, M.E. & Mahalik, J.R. (2003) Men, masculinity, and the contexts of help seeking. *American Psychologist*, **58**, 5–14.

Albertson, P. (1997) Prostate disease in older men: cancer. *Hospital Practice*, **32**(10), 159–166, 171, 175–176.

Aneshensel, C.S., Estrada, A.L., Hansell, M.J. & Clark, V.A. (1987) Social psychological aspects of reporting behavior: lifetime depressive episode reports. *Journal of Health and Social Behavior*, **28**, 232–246.

Angst, J., Gamma, A., Gastpar, M., Lépine, J-P., Mendlewicz, J. & Tylee, A. (2002) Gender differences in depression: epidemiological findings from the European DEPRES I and II studies. *European Archives of Psychiatry and Clinical Neuroscience*, **252**, 201–209.

Arrington, M. (2003) 'I don't want to be an artificial man': narrative reconstruction of sexuality among prostate cancer survivors. *Sexuality and Culture*, **7**(2), 30–58.

Aucoin, M.W. & Wassersug, R.J. (2006) The sexuality and social performance of androgen-deprived (castrated men) throughout history: implications for modern day cancer patients. *Social Science and Medicine*, **63**(12), 3162–3173.

Banks, I. (2001) No man's land: men, illness and the NHS. *British Medical Journal*, **323**, 1058–1060.

Baquet, C.R., Horm, J.W., Gibbs, T. & Greenwald, P. (1991) Socioeconomic factors and cancer incidence among blacks and whites. *Journal of the National Cancer Institute*, **83**, 551–557.

Boring, C.C., Squires, T.S. & Heath, C.W. Jr. (1992) Cancer statistics for African Americans. *CA: A Cancer Journal for Clinicians*, **42**, 7–17.

Bottorff, J.L., Oliffe, J.L., Halpin, M., Phillips, M., McLean, G. & Mroz, L. (2008). Women and prostate cancer support groups: the gender connect? *Social Science and Medicine*, **66**(5), 1217–1227.

Broom, A. (2004) Prostate cancer and masculinity in Australian society: a case of stolen identity? *International Journal of Men's Health*, **3**(2), 73–91.

Broom, A. (2005a) Medical specialists' accounts of the impact of the internet on the doctor/patient relationship. *Health*, **9**(3), 319–338.

Broom, A. (2005b) The eMale: prostate cancer, masculinity and online support as a challenge to medical expertise. *Journal of Sociology*, **41**(1), 87–104.

Broom, A. (2005c) Virtually healthy: the impact of internet use on disease experience and the doctor–patient relationship. *Qualitative Health Research*, **15**(3), 325–345.

Cancer Council Australia (2007) *National Cancer Prevention Policy 2007–2009*, pp.164–175. NSW: Cancer Council Australia.

Chan, E.C.Y. & Sulmay, D.P. (1998) What men should know about prostate-specific antigen screening before giving informed consent? *American Journal of Medicine*, **105**, 266–274.

Chapple, A. & Ziebland, S. (2002) Prostate cancer: embodied experience and perceptions of masculinity. *Sociology of Health & Illness*, **24**(6), 820–841.

Chapple, A.B., Ziebland, S., Brewster, S. & McPherson, A. (2007) Patients' perceptions of transrectal prostate biopsy: a qualitative study. *European Journal of Cancer Care*, **16**(3), 215–221.

Charmaz, K. (1995) Identity, dilemmas of chronically ill men. In: *Men's Health and Illness: Gender, Power and the Body* (eds D. Sabo & D.F. Gordon), pp.266–291. Thousand Oaks, CA: Sage Publications.

Connell, R.W. (1995) *Masculinities*. Berkeley, CA: University of California Press.

Courtenay, W.H. (1998) College men's health: an overview and a call to action. *Journal of American College Health*, **46**, 279–290.

Courtenay, W.H. (2000) Constructions of masculinity and their influence on men's well-being: a theory of gender and health. *Social Science and Medicine*, **50**(10), 1385–1401.

Courtenay, W.H. (2004) Best practices for improving college men's health. *New Directions for Student Services*, **107**, 59–74.

Dale, W., Sartor, S., Davis, T. & Bennett, C.L. (1999) Understanding barriers to the elderly detection of prostate cancer among men of lower socioeconomic status. *Prostate Journal*, **1**(4), 179–184.

Dunn, I.B. & Kirk, D. (2000) Legal pitfalls in the diagnosis of prostate cancer. *British Journal of Urology International*, **86**, 304–307.

Edgar, D. (1997) *Men, Mateship, Marriage*. Pymble, New South Wales: Harper Collins.

Fergus, K.D., Gray, R.E. & Fitch, M.I. (2002) Sexual dysfunction and the preservation of manhood: experiences of men with prostate cancer. *Journal of Health Psychology*, **7**(3), 303–316.

Forrester-Anderson, I.T. (2005) Prostate cancer screening perceptions, knowledge, and behaviors among African American men: focus group findings. *Journal of Health Care for the Poor and Underserved*, **16**(4), Suppl. A, 22–30.

Frank, B., Numer, M., Evans, J., Oliffe, J.L., Devine, D. & Gregory, D. (2007) A framework for Health, Illness, Men and Masculinities (HIMM). *Journal of Men's Health and Gender*, **4**(3), 358–359.

Galdas, P.M., Cheater, F. & Marshall, P. (2005) Men and health help-seeking behaviour: literature review. *Journal of Advanced Nursing*, **49**(6), 616–623.

Gorman, C. (2002) What's a guy to do? Most men who get tested don't die from it. So why get tested? Good question. *Time*, **159**(11), 98.

Gray, R.E. (2003) *Prostate Tales: Men's Experiences with Prostate Cancer*. Harriman, TN: Men's Studies Press.

Gray, R.E. & Klotz, L.H. (2004) Restoring sexual function in prostate cancer patients: an innovative approach. *Canadian Journal of Urology*, **11**(3), 2285–2289.

Gray, R.E., Fitch, M.I., Fergus, K.D., Mykhalovskiy, E. & Church, K. (2002) Hegemonic masculinity and the experience of prostate cancer: a narrative approach. *Journal of Aging and Identity*, **7**(1), 43–62.

Gray, R.E., Wassersug, R.J., Sinding, C., Barbara, A.M., Trosztmer, C. & Fleshner, N. (2005) The experiences of men receiving androgen deprivation treatment for prostate cancer: a qualitative study. *Canadian Journal of Urology*, **12**(4), 2755–2763.

Grossman, M. & Wood, W. (1993) Sex differences in intensity of emotional experience: a social role interpretation. *Journal of Personality and Social Psychology*, **65**(5), 1010–1022.

Haas, G.P., Montie, J. & Pontes, J.E. (1993) The state of prostate cancer screening in the United States. *European Urology*, **23**, 337–347.

Hayes, R. (2001) Gender distinctions but not gender dissociations. In: *Women's Health/ Men's Health Working Together? Proceedings of Women's Health Victoria's Forum* (eds S. Brown & R. Bachowski), pp.8–15. Melbourne, Australia: Women's Health Victoria.

Heesacker, M., Wester, S.R., Vogel, D.L., Wentzel, J.T., Mejia-Millan, C.M. & Gooholm, C.R. (1999) Gender-based emotional stereotyping. *Journal of Counseling Psychology*, **46**(4), 483–495.

Hirst, G., Ward, J. & Del Mar, C. (1996) Prostate cancer screening: the case against. *Medical Journal of Australia*, **164**, 285–287.

Honkalampi, K., Saarinen, P., Hintikka, J., Virtanen, V. & Viinamaki, H. (1999) Factors associated with alexithymia in patients suffering from depression. *Psychotherapy and Psychosomatics*, **68**, 270–275.

Hsing, A.W., Tsao, L. & Devesa, S.S. (2000) International trends and patterns of prostate cancer incidence and mortality. *International Journal of Cancer*, **85**(1), 60–67.

Jemal, A., Siegel, R., Ward, E., Murray, T., Xu, J. & Thun, M.J. (2007) Cancer statistics. *CA. A Cancer Journal for Clinicians*, **57**, 43–66.

Jones, J. (1996) *Understanding of health: the background to a study of rural men's perceptions of health.* Paper presented at the 3rd Biennial Australian Rural and Remote Health Science Conference, August, Toowoomba, Queensland, Australia.

Kim, L. (2000) Gel greatly reduces prostate biopsy pain. *Emory Report*, **52**(37), (Online). Available at: http://www.emory.edu/EMORY_REPORT/erarchive/ 2000/July/erjuly. 10/7_10_00prostate.html

Kimmel, M. (1994) Masculinities as homophobia: fear, shame, and silence in the construction of gender identity. In: *Theorizing Masculinities* (eds H. Brod & M. Kaufman), pp.119–141. Thousand Oaks, CA: Sage Publications.

Kozlowski, J. & Grayhack, J. (2002) Carcinoma of the prostate. In: *Adult and Pediatric Urology*, Vol. 2 (eds J. Gillenwater, J. Grayhack, S. Howards & M. Mitchell), 4th edn. pp.1471–1654. Philadelphia, PA: Lippincott Williams & Williams.

Laws, T., Drummond, M. & Polijak-Fligic, J. (2000) On what basis do Australian men make informed decisions about diagnostic and treatment options for prostate cancer? *Australian Journal of Primary Health – Interchange*, **6**(2), 86–93.

Lee, C. & Owens, R. (2002) *The Psychology of Men's Health Series.* Philadelphia, PA: Open University Press.

Lohan, M. (2007) How might we understand men's health better? Integrating explanations from critical studies on men and inequalities in health. *Social Science and Medicine*, **65**(3), 493–504.

Macias, D.J., Sarabia, M.J. & Sklar, D.P. (2000) Male discomfort during digital rectal examination: does examiner gender make a difference? *American Journal of Emergency Medicine*, **18**(6), 676–678.

Mahalik, J.R., Locke, B.D., Ludlow, L.H. et al. (2003) Development of the conformity to Masculine Norms Inventory. *Journal of Men and Masculinity*, **4**, 3–25.

Mansfield, A.K., Addis, M.E. & Mahalik, J.R. (2003) Why won't he go to the doctor? The psychology of men's help-seeking. *International Journal of Men's Health*, **2**(2), 93–110.

Martino, W. & Pallotta-Chiarolli, M. (2003) *So What's a Boy? Addressing Issues of Masculinity and Schooling.* Maidenhead, UK: Open University Press.

Moynihan, C. (1998) Theories in health care in research: theories of masculinity. *British Medical Journal*, **317**, 1072–1075.

Nagler, H., Gerber, E., Homel, P. et al. (2005) Digital rectal examination is barrier to population-based prostate cancer screening. *Urology*, **65**(6), 1137–1140.

Navon, L. & Morag, A. (2003a) Advanced prostate cancer patients' relationships with their spouses following hormonal therapy. *European Journal of Oncology Nursing,* 7(2), 73–80.

Navon, L. & Morag, A. (2003b) Advanced prostate cancer patients' ways of coping with the hormonal therapy's effect on body, sexuality, and spousal ties. *Qualitative Health Research,* **13**(10), 1378–1392.

Navon, L. & Morag, A. (2004) Liminality as biographical disruption: unclassifiability following hormonal therapy for advanced prostate cancer. *Social Science and Medicine,* **58**(11), 2337–2347.

O'Brien, R., Hunt, K. & Hart, G. (2005) 'It's caveman stuff, but that is to a certain extent how guys still operate': men's accounts of masculinity and help seeking. *Social Science and Medicine,* **61**(3), 503–516.

O'Hehir, B., Scotney, E. & Anderson, G. (1997) *Healthy lifestyles: are rural men getting the message?* Paper presented at the National Rural Health Forum: Rural Public Health in Australia, June, Adelaide, Australia.

Oliffe, J.L. (2002) In search of a social model of prostate cancer: finding out about Bronch. In: *Manning the Next Millennium: Studies in Masculinities* (eds S. Pearce & V. Muller), pp.69–84. Western Australia: Black Swan Press.

Oliffe, J.L. (2003) *Prostate cancer: Anglo-Australian heterosexual perspectives* (Dissertation). Available at: http://tux.lib.deakin.edu.au/adt-VDU/public/adt-VDU20050712.095519/

Oliffe, J.L. (2004a) Anglo-Australian masculinities and trans rectal ultrasound prostate biopsy (TRUS-Bx): connections and collisions. *International Journal of Men's Health,* **3**(1), 43–60.

Oliffe, J.L. (2004b) Transrectal ultrasound prostate biopsy (TRUS-Bx): patient perspectives. *Urologic Nursing,* **24**(5), 395–400.

Oliffe, J.L. (2005) Constructions of masculinity following prostatectomy-induced impotence. *Social Science and Medicine,* **60**(10), 2240–2259.

Oliffe, J.L. (2006a) Being screened for prostate cancer: a simple blood test or a commitment to treatment? *Cancer Nursing,* **29**(1), 1–8.

Oliffe, J.L. (2006b) Embodied masculinity and androgen deprivation therapy. *Sociology of Health and Illness,* **28**(4), 410–432.

Oliffe, J.L. (in press) Health behaviors, prostate cancer and masculinities: a life course perspective. *Men and Masculinities.*

Oliffe, J.L. & Bottorff, J.L. (2006) Men's health and ethnography. *Journal of Men's Health and Gender,* **3**(1), 104–108.

Oliffe, J.L. & Thorne, S.E. (2007) Men, masculinities and prostate cancer: Australian and Canadian patient perspectives of communication with male physicians. *Qualitative Health Research,* **17**(2), 149–161.

Oliffe, J.L., Halpin, M., Bottorff, J.L., Hislop, T.G., McKenzie, M. & Mroz, L. (2008). How prostate cancer support groups do and do not survive: British Columbian perspectives. *American Journal of Men's Health,* **2**(2), 143–155.

Oliffe, J.L., Davison, B.J., Pickles, T. & Mroz, L. (in press). Self-management of uncertainty in active surveillence. *Qualitative Health Research.*

Parkin, D. (2001) Global cancer statistics in the year 2000. *Lancet Oncology,* **2**(9), 533–543.

Parkin, D.M., Bray, F.I. & Devesa, S.S. (2001) Cancer burden in the year 2000: the global picture. *European Journal of Cancer,* **37**, Suppl. 8, 4–66.

Pescorosolido, B.A. & Boyer, C.A. (1999) How do people come to use mental health services? Current knowledge and changing perspectives. In: *A Handbook for the Study of Mental Health: Social Context, Theories and Systems* (eds A.V. Horwitz & T.L. Scheid), pp.392–411. New York: Cambridge University Press.

Pickles, T., Ruether, J.D., Weir, L., Carlson, L. & Jakulj, F. (2007) Psychosocial barriers to active surveillance for the management of early prostate cancer and a strategy for increased acceptance. *BJU International*, online, retrieved 5 July 2007.

Pinnock, C., O'Brien, B.O. & Marshall, V.R. (1998) Older men's concerns about their urological health: a qualitative study. *Australian and New Zealand Journal of Public Health*, **22**(3), 368–373.

Potts, A. (2000) The essence of the hard-on: hegemonic masculinity and the cultural construction of 'erectile dysfunction'. *Men and Masculinities*, **3**(1), 85–103.

Potts, A., Gavey, N., Grace, V.M. & Vares, T. (2003) The downside of Viagra: women's experiences and concerns. *Sociology of Health and Illness*, **25**(7), 697–719.

Potts, A., Grace, V., Gavey, N. & Vares, T. (2004) 'Viagra stories': challenging 'erectile dysfunction'. *Social Science and Medicine*, **59**, 489–499.

Quinn, M. & Babb, P. (2002a) Patterns and trends in prostate cancer incidence, survival, prevalence and mortality. Part I: international comparisons. *British Journal of Urology International*, **90**, 162–173.

Quinn, M. & Babb, P. (2002b) Patterns and trends in prostate cancer incidence, survival, prevalence and mortality. Part II: individual countries. *British Journal of Urology International*, **90**, 174–184.

Robertson, S. (2003) Men managing health. *Men's Health Journal*, **2**(4), 111–113.

Robertson, S. (2007) *Understanding Men and Health Masculinities, Identity and Wellbeing.* Maidenhead, UK: Open University Press.

Seymour-Smith, S., Wetherell, M. & Phoenix, A. (2002) 'My wife ordered me to come!': A discursive analysis of doctors' and nurses' accounts of men's use of general practitioners. *Journal of Health Psychology*, **7**(3), 253–267.

Smith, D.P., Armstrong, B.K. & Saunders, R. (1998) *Patterns of Prostate Specific Antigen (PSA) Testing in Australia in 1992 to 1996: An Examination of Medicare Data.* Sydney, Australia: New South Wales Cancer Council.

Taylor, C., Stewart, A. & Parker, R. (1998) 'Machismo' as the barrier to health promotion in Australian males. In: *Promoting Men's Health – An Essential Book for Nurses* (ed. T. Laws), pp.15–30. Melbourne: Ausmed Publications.

Taylor, J.S. (1993) Carcinoma of the prostate. *Medical Journal of Australia*, **159**, 436–437.

Tiefer, L. (1987) In pursuit of the perfect penis: the medicalisation of male sexuality. In: *Changing Men: New Directions in Research on Men and Masculinity* (ed. M. Kimmel), pp.579–599. Newbury, CA: Sage Publications.

United Nations (2007) *World population ageing 2007: executive summary* (Online). Available at: http://www.un.org/esa/population/publications/WPA2007/wpp2007.htm

Vilas, S. (2003) *Masculinity versus Castration: On the Way to Fighting Prostate Cancer.* Baton Rouge, LA: Yago Editorial LLC.

Ward, J.E., Gupta, L. & Taylor, N.J. (1998) Do general practitioners use prostate-specific antigen as a screening test for early prostate cancer? *Medical Journal of Australia*, **169**, 29–31.

Warkentin, K.M., Gray, R.E. & Wassersug, R.J. (2006) Restoration of satisfying sex for a castrated cancer patient with complete impotence: a case study. *Journal of Sex and Marital Therapy*, **32**, 389–399.

Wassersug, R.J. (in press) Mastering emasculation. *Journal of Clinical Oncology*.

Wassersug, R.J. & Johnson, T.W. (2007) Modern-day eunuchs: motivations for and consequences of contemporary castration. *Perspectives in Biology and Medicine*, **50**(4), 544–556.

Wassersug, R.J. & Oliffe, J.L. (in press) On the meaning of gynecomastia to men, women, and the medical community. *Journal of Sexual Medicine*.

Watson, J. (2000) *Male Bodies: Health, Culture and Identity*. Philadelphia, PA: Open Press.

White, A. (2001) How men respond to illness. *Men's Health Journal*, **1**(1), 18–19.

White, P., Young, K. & McTeer, W. (1995) Sports, masculinity, and the injured body. In *Men's Health and Illness: Gender, Power and the Body* (eds D. Suso & F. Gordon), pp.158–182. Thousand Oaks, CA: Sage Publications.

Wilhelm, K., Roy, K., Mitchell, P., Brownhill, S. & Parker, G. (2002) Gender differences in depression risk and coping factors in a clinical sample. *Acta Psychiatrica Scandinavica*, **106**, 45–53.

Ziguras, C. (1998) Masculinity and self-care. In: *Promoting Men's Health: An Essential Book for Nurses* (ed. T. Laws), pp.45–61. Melbourne: Ausmed Publications.

Zisman, A., Leibovici, D., Siegel, Y. & Lindner, A. (1999) Complications and quality of life impairment after ultrasound guided prostate biopsy: a prospective study. *Cancer Weekly Plus*, August, **9**(3).

Zisman, A., Leibovici, D., Siegel, Y. & Lindner, A. (2001) The impact of prostate biopsy on patient well-being: a prospective study of pain, anxiety and erectile dysfunction. *Journal of Urology*, **165**(2), 445–454.

# Chapter 3

# MEN, MASCULINITY AND HELP-SEEKING BEHAVIOUR

Paul M. Galdas

## Introduction

Popular stereotypes have long characterised men as unwilling to ask for help, so it is perhaps unsurprising that the rapid growth in interest in men's health studies has seen a corresponding interest in men's health-related help-seeking behaviour. Over the past decade, numerous researchers and authors have studied and provided commentary on men's apparent failure to engage with preventive healthcare and health promotion, their poor awareness of their bodies and the symptoms of ill-health, and their reticence to seek and utilise acute healthcare services in a timely manner when experiencing various physical and emotional problems. This chapter sets out to critically examine the research knowledge in this emerging field of men's health in order to illuminate whether there is a sufficient evidence-base to support popular stereotypes of men as reluctant healthcare seekers, and, if so, why this might be the case.

The key theoretical processes in relation to intersections between masculinities and men's help-seeking behaviour are discussed with regard to the efficacy and limitations of current empirical evidence. Particular attention is paid to the body of literature that has explored how representations of culturally dominant versions of (hegemonic) masculinity intersect with men's health-related help-seeking practices. Focus is drawn to some of the most recent and original work in the field in order to illustrate the need to move beyond examining men's help-seeking with an essentialist hegemonic analytical lens, toward a more inclusive gender framework that recognises the composite, fluid and contextually dependent nature of men's masculine constructions and their impact on health-related help-seeking practices.

## Are men more reluctant to seek help than women, or is it just a myth?

The possibility that poor health-related behaviour on the part of men might account for the disparity between men's and women's rates of mortality and morbidity was raised as early as the mid-1970s (Waldron, 1976; Harrison, 1978). However, as indicated in Chapter 1, men's help-seeking behaviour has only recently come to be considered problematic (Courtenay, 2000). The issue of 'help-seeking' can broadly be considered to be concerned with how individuals become aware of, and respond to, health concerns or the symptoms of ill-health against the background of social norms and cultural practices (Smith et al., 2006). In the past, men's rates of help-seeking for health problems had largely been considered to be normative; evidence of men's lower incidence of healthcare utilisation compared to women has often been explained as being an artefact of women's over-utilisation of services (Courtenay, 2000). However, in the past decade numerous sources have recognised that men may indeed be less likely than women to seek help for comparable health-related problems, and since early detection is often critical for preventing disease and death, men's reticence to seek medical help in a timely manner may have profound consequences for their health. Subsequent ministers for public health in the United Kingdom have, for instance, openly highlighted men's help-seeking behaviour as a significant public health issue. Specifically, ministers have noted that 'men are less likely [than women] to visit a doctor when they are ill and are less likely to report on the symptoms of disease or illness' (Department of Health, 2000) and that 'traditional male attitudes' can have an adverse impact on men's health, in particular, 'being independent', 'not asking for help', and 'being self-contained' (Health Development Agency, 2002). The president of the Men's Health Forum has argued that men's 'apparent reluctance to consult a doctor' has made health services a 'no man's land' (Banks, 2001, p.1058) and a scoping study of key individuals and organisations that have a role in the care of men in the UK has also revealed a reluctance to access health services as the principal issue facing men's health (White, 2001). This political and professional interest has placed help-seeking behaviour at the forefront of the men's health research agenda. The following quote, taken from a study of US physicians' perspectives of men's help-seeking behaviour, reflects the motivation for much of the recent surge in interest:

*The literature describes a relative under use of health care services by men despite the fact men are susceptible to particular types of illness and disease. Men are less likely than women to actively seek medical care when they are ill, choosing instead to 'tough it out'... possibly decreasing their chance for early detection, treatment and even prevention of disease.* (Tudiver & Talbot, 1999, p.47)

However, a review of the research literature addressing men's and women's patterns of help-seeking behaviour and healthcare utilisation reveals a more intricate picture than popular stereotypes and the above quote might suggest.

The empirical origins of the supposition that men seek and utilise healthcare and medical services less than women (as opposed to women over-utilising services) originate primarily from the findings of several studies that examined differences in the frequency with which men and women sought help for a range of health problems (Courtenay, 2002; Addis & Mahalik, 2003). Several studies in the US indicated that men were less likely than women to seek help from healthcare professionals for problems as diverse as depression, substance abuse, physical disabilities and stressful life events (Weissman & Klerman, 1977; Padesky & Hammen, 1981; Thom, 1986; Husaini et al., 1994; McKay et al., 1996; Courtenay, 2002). With regard to physical health, evidence from the US and UK has also shown that men use primary healthcare services (and general practitioners in particular) to a lesser extent than their female counterparts. Cook et al. (1990) found that across all social classes, 10% of men aged 45–65 in the UK did not consult their general practitioner (GP) over a three-year period, and a further 44% consulted on average twice a year or less. Similar findings have been reported in a survey study which found 69% of men in the UK aged 18–24 had visited their family physician's surgery in the preceding 12 months compared with 90% of women of the same age group; and furthermore only 58% of men in excellent health attended their surgery compared with 74% of women, suggesting men were also poor attendees for preventive medicine (NHS Executive, 1998).

Other studies have indicated that men not only seek medical help less often than women, but their reasons for doing so also differ. Although minor emotional symptoms increase the probability of consulting a GP, physical symptoms have been shown to be the determining factor for men seeking help (Möller-Leimkühler, 2002). In contrast to women, it has also been shown that men do not report psychosocial problems and distress as an additional reason for consulting their GP (Corney, 1990). Men's lower rates of treatment for depressive symptoms compared to women have thus been suggested as being attributable to gender-related discrepancies in perception of need and help-seeking behaviour (Möller-Leimkühler, 2002).

These, and other similar studies, have led many commentators to conclude that there is 'overwhelming' evidence that men are more reticent to seek medical help and utilise healthcare services compared to women (Courtenay, 2002; Addis & Mahalik, 2003; Men's Health Forum, 2004; Mansfield et al., 2005; Smith et al. 2006; White et al., 2006). However, evidence highlighting delays in *women's* help-seeking has led some to challenge this assertion and, in doing so, have inadvertently highlighted a fundamental limitation of sex-disaggregated data on help-seeking behaviour (Macintyre et al., 1996). The literature on the influence of sex and/or gender on help-seeking for the symptoms of myocardial infarction (heart attack) is a case in point. Recognition that the most critical factor in preventing premature death from myocardial infarction is the delivery of prompt medical treatment (e.g. GISSI, 1986, 1995; ISIS-2, 1988; UKHAS, 1998) indicates that any delay in help-seeking when a myocardial infarction is suspected is problematic, and a review of the research literature highlights this as a long-recognised problem (White & Johnson, 2000; Emslie, 2005). Yet despite coronary heart disease being the leading cause of premature death for men worldwide, a recent systematic review of studies investigating the predictors of delay in seeking medical help in patients with suspected myocardial infarction indicated that *females* delay seeking help significantly longer than males (Hewitt et al., 2004). Similarly, a qualitative synthesis of studies exploring patients' help-seeking experiences and delay in cancer presentation identified women as frequent help-seeking delayers because they prioritised work and family responsibilities over their own health (Smith et al., 2005).

In light of this evidence, are we to conclude that hypotheses about men being more disinclined to seek help than women are merely myths? That medical help-seeking is actually a women's health issue in the context of heart disease and cancer? Or that help-seeking behaviour is not a gender issue at all? By searching for an answer to this question, as many researchers continue to do, the principle rationale for studying sex and gender in relation to help-seeking behaviour is at risk of being overlooked. To illustrate this argument by returning to the example of heart disease: understanding sex differences might be a starting point for teasing out men's and women's differing help-seeking behavioural patterns when they experience myocardial infarction, but sex-based binary comparisons do little to help inform the development of healthcare interventions, practice or policy that will better engage men with healthcare services when they suffer an acute cardiac event. Of greater relevance than evidence about which sex is the greater 'delayer' is knowledge about gender-specific processes that underlie men's (and women's) decision-making and resulting help-seeking behaviour when they experience the symptoms of a heart attack. The same can be argued for all sex comparative help-seeking studies; that is, the fact that men and women might differ in the frequency of a set of behaviours reveals little about the gender-related processes responsible for any observed differences (Mechanic, 1978). As Addis and Mahalik (2003) have pointed out, when studies have documented sex differences the authors have often speculated about possible mediators of help-seeking behaviour, but rarely have the data been able to address directly the gender-specific reasons for the delays. Rather, most studies exploring differences in male and female help-seeking behaviour have reduced sex or gender to quantitative differences in research variables (Möller-Leimkühler, 2002). Another criticism of sex-difference studies is a general one, applying to all approaches of this kind. Binary comparisons between men's and women's help-seeking behaviours also serve to obscure significant differences *among* men – based on factors such as age, sexuality, socioeconomic status, culture and ethnicity – that may be greater than the observed behavioural differences *between* men and women. Research is beginning to show that relative under-utilisation of healthcare services is not a uniform phenomenon for all men. As discussed later in this chapter, for instance, there is evidence that men of differing ethnicity seek medical help for the symptoms of an acute cardiac event within different time intervals and for different reasons, which may limit their opportunity for particular interventions or outcomes, and which require gender culturally sensitive interventions. In order to understand why some groups of men may have difficulty in seeking and accessing medical help and how gender intersects with their help-seeking decision-making, it is necessary to focus investigations on *men's* experiences of seeking help, not merely on sex-disaggregated data and the superficial differences between men's and women's patterns of behaviour. It is on this body of knowledge that the remainder of this chapter will focus.

## Gender role socialisation and help-seeking behaviour

Critiquing the research knowledge on men, masculinity and help-seeking behaviour has been made complex by variations in how gender has been understood and conceptualised by social scientists and men's health researchers. One approach that has been widely used for understanding men's orientation to seeking medical help has been masculine/male gender-role socialisation theories. The approach begins with the theoretical premise that men and women learn gendered attitudes and behaviours from cultural values, norms and ideologies about what it means to be men and women (Addis & Mahalik, 2003) and has most commonly been exhibited in investigations into the deleterious impact of 'gender role conflict' (a psychological state where gender roles have negative consequences or impact on a person or others) and 'masculine ideology' (an individual's endorsement and internalisation of cultural norms and values regarding masculinity and the male role) on men's health (Pleck et al., 1994; Addis & Mahalik, 2003; Mansfield et al., 2003). Harrison and colleagues (1989, p.271) explain:

> ... the greater mortality rate of men is at least partially a consequence of the demands of the male role and emphasizes the ways in which male-role expectations have a deleterious effect on men's lives, and possibly contribute to men's higher mortality rate.

Male role expectations, or gender role conflict, have been theorised to have a number of damaging effects on men's health behaviours. For example, taking a 'give 'em hell' approach to life – the need to be more powerful than others, through violence if necessary (Brannon, 1976) – has been theorised to lead to high-risk behaviours (Sabo & Gordon, 1995). Similarly, recognising and labelling an emotional problem and admitting a need for medical help has been suggested to conflict with the messages men receive about the importance of self-reliance, physical toughness and emotional control (Pleck, 1981; Addis & Mahalik, 2003).

Several studies have employed this framework in testing (usually quantitatively) the relationship between gender role conflict/masculine ideologies and men's attitudes toward help-seeking. For instance, in one study of the health beliefs and attitudes of a group of healthy 25- to 35-year-old men, most were found to have ignored symptoms of ill-health and avoided seeking help from health services in the past (Sharpe & Arnold, 1998). Results revealed that a majority of men agreed that 'minor illness can be fought off if you don't give in to it' (64%); 'I often ignore symptoms hoping they will go away' (52%); and 'I have to be really ill before I go and see the doctor' (75%). This, the researchers argued, reinforced theories that a traditional masculine gender role has a damaging influence on men's health. In a more general, and perhaps typical, study in this literature, Good and colleagues (1989) set out to test the hypothesis that adherence to a traditional male gender role and negative attitudes to help-seeking were related, using a sample drawn from undergraduate university students. Subjects were asked to complete stereotypical male role and gender role conflict measures associated with factors such as success, power, competition and avoiding emotional expression ('restrictive emotionality'). The findings showed that traditional attitudes about the male role were significantly linked to negative attitudes toward seeking professional help. Those who were found to have 'restrictive emotionality' were also identified as having significantly decreased past help-seeking behaviour and decreased likelihood of future help-seeking behaviour.

Addis and Mahalik (2003) have argued that these and other similar empirical investigations (for example, Helgeson, 1995; Mendoza & Cummings, 2001; McCarthy & Holliday, 2004) show that male-gender role socialisation theory has direct clinical relevance to men's help-seeking, such as in the treatment of depression. However, a significant and frequently overlooked limitation of this body of evidence is the cultural assumptions and expectations evident in the studies' methodologies that pre-empt static responses which serve to perpetuate the myth of what it means to be masculine, how a man behaves, and also what constitutes traditional or dominant masculine practice in contemporary western society (Moynihan, 1998). Akin to the sex differences approach, male gender role studies have thus failed to adequately address variability among differing groups of men; a flaw that has been compounded by the repeated use of samples of white, heterosexual, middle-class males.

Recent qualitative research is increasingly revealing the complex nature of masculinities and how they interplay with men's health behaviours in various social contexts; illustrating among other things that not all men consider 'traditional masculine ideologies' to be central to their masculine identity or important in their experience of seeking medical help. Yet, quantitative instruments based on a gender role socialisation paradigm[1] necessitate men to rate their endorsement of static, simplistic (and perhaps outdated) ideologies such as self-reliance, competitiveness, power over others, and aggression, without any observation of men's actual behaviour or gender practices (Hearn, 1994). In the case of Sharpe and Arnold's (1998) study, for example, their data provides no explanation of why 48% of their subjects did not agree with the statement 'I often ignore symptoms hoping they will go away' or how these men may have represented their masculinity in the context of seeking medical help. To answer this question, and gain a more fluid, in-depth insight into the key masculine processes at work in the context of men's help-seeking behaviour, it is necessary to move away from heavy dependence on quantitative variables that categorise men's gendered experiences and render them as uniform, toward

---

[1] Including commonly used inventories such as the Bem sex role inventory (BSRI) (Bem, 1974), the personal attributes questionnaire (PAQ) (Spence et al., 1974) and masculine gender role stress scale (MGRS) (Eisler & Skidmore, 1987).

qualitative data that explicitly addresses how masculinities are *socially constructed* in the context of seeking medical help.

## Help-seeking vis-à-vis the social construction of hegemonic masculinity

In the social constructionist paradigm, men's help-seeking behaviour is considered to be a social act which constructs 'the person' in the same way that other social and cultural activities do. That is, health-related behaviours – such as seeking medical help – can (and are) used by men as a representation of masculinity akin to those constructed in the work environment or sporting arena. Accordingly, health behaviours are an opportunity for men to demonstrate 'real' manhood to themselves and others (Saltonstall, 1993; Courtenay, 2000). Courtenay (2000) powerfully explains this premise in his frequently quoted hypothesis, as discussed in Chapter 1, that a man who 'does' masculinity as socially prescribed (in western culture) would be relatively unconcerned about his health and wellbeing in general, place little value on health knowledge, think of himself as independent and not needing to be nurtured by others. The relevance of this in the context of help-seeking, as Courtenay (2000) goes on to explain, is that when a man brags 'I haven't been to a doctor in years', he is simultaneously describing a health practice and situating himself in a masculine arena.

The concept of hegemonic masculinity has dominated recent constructionist examinations into how gender intersects with men's health-related help-seeking practices (Connell & Messerschmidt, 2005). As outlined in this text's introduction, hegemonic masculinity refers to the most honoured, desired and culturally authoritative form of masculinity in any given context and is seen as the representation of gender practice that sets the standards for all other men and against which other men are measured (Kimmel, 1996; Connell, 2000, 2005; Connell & Messerschmidt, 2005). The fear of marginalisation – being seen as weak or inadequate as a man – dominates western definitions of manhood (Kimmel 1996; Connell, 2005), and men's subsequent desire to 'live up' to the dominant, hegemonic masculine ideal has often been theorised to impinge on them in real and problematic ways; most notably, with respect to their help-seeking behaviour and reticence to utilise healthcare services. Men may face risk and physical discomfort rather than transgress social expectations for male gender-appropriate help-seeking behaviour and be associated with (emasculating) traits such as vulnerability, dependence and weakness (Courtenay, 2000; Lee & Owens, 2002; Mansfield et al., 2003).

Empirical data are increasingly bearing out these theorised connections between hegemonic masculinity and men's poor help-seeking practices. In particular, several studies have implicated hegemonic masculinity as having a detrimental effect on how men manage the impact of prostate cancer on their life, specifically in relation to expressing emotion and seeking emotional support. For example, Gray and colleagues (2000) implicated hegemonic forms of masculinity as having a detrimental effect on how men with prostate cancer expressed emotion and sought emotional support, which in turn impacted on their relationships, the ability to manage their feelings, the ability to make sense of their illness, and the ability to lessen the impact the cancer had on their everyday lives (Gray et al., 2000). Broom (2004) interviewed 33 Australian men with prostate cancer and also found that because of many men's desire to adhere to hegemonic forms of masculinity, the nature and effect of investigative, diagnostic and treatment procedures for prostate cancer – incontinence, loss of potency and transrectal examination – led many to choose to forgo these treatments as they prioritised aspects of their lifestyle (associated with hegemonic masculinity) over 'best' chance of cure.

In perhaps one of the most interesting studies in the prostate cancer literature, Evans and colleagues (2005) studied the experiences of 57 African Canadian men diagnosed with prostate cancer in Nova Scotia, Canada – an investigation noteworthy because it is one of the few in the men's health literature that has examined gender representations among men from a minority ethnic group. Yet, despite their unique study sample, the themes identified cohered with those described by Broom (2004) and others: upholding a dominant masculine identity was reported as a critical factor in men's avoidance of cancer screening, especially digital rectal examination (DRE). This, the researchers argued, showed that:

> ...because historically, Black men have not been rewarded for being manly, courageous, or assertive – a situation that has stripped Black men of their masculinity... avenues for demonstrating masculinity are narrowed for Black men such that sexual virility and sexual performance may be the primary ways that African Nova Scotian men can affirm their identity as a man... Black men's practices of avoiding DREs may consequently be understood as practices to protect and defend an already compromised masculinity. (Evans et al., 2005, p.268)

Although Evans et al.'s (2005) findings provide a rare insight into the gendered experiences of black Afro-Canadian men with prostate cancer, the main findings in this study may in fact point toward commonalities between men of a similar age as opposed to variation between men of differing race or ethnicity. Related findings in studies of white participants by George and Fleming (2004), Boehmer and Clark (2001) and Broom (2004) would suggest that sexual performance, sexual virility and the avoidance of DRE are key aspects of constructing or preserving young men's masculinity, regardless of their ethnicity. One study, based on a sample of white men diagnosed with prostate cancer in the UK, makes this point clear. Chapple and Ziebland (2002) investigated the way in which prostate cancer and its treatment affected men's bodies, their roles and sense of masculinity. The principal findings illustrated that men were hesitant about seeking help for their problems because they believed it was not 'macho' to seek advice about health problems, that 'boys don't cry', and it was not 'masculine' to display signs of weakness (Chapple & Ziebland, 2002). This echoes the narratives of African Canadian men in Evans et al.'s (2005) study who had been reluctant to share their cancer experience with others because, as one participant in the study pointed out, 'I don't want people to know I am a weakling' (p.265).

Similar stories of a reluctance to seek or admit the need for medical help have been told by white or European men with testicular cancer (Moynihan, 1998; Gascoigne & Whitear, 1999; Chapple et al., 2004; Mason & Strauss, 2004; Smith et al., 2005) and men seeking help for the symptoms of an acute cardiac event (White, 2000). White (2000) has provided a particularly interesting account of the link between the social construction of 'masculinity' and help-seeking delays, arguing that men are continually undergoing self-surveillance to assess their performance against their impressions of society's expectations of them; a performance which is threatened by the possibility of ill-health and leads to the use of denial as a psychological defence and, therefore, a reluctance to seek help:

> It seems that man [sic] is not prepared to deal with his body when it makes the transition from being healthy to being ill. He is expected to be fit, productive and able to carry out the roles expected of him. There is a feeling of invincibility that is deep seated and, when this is threatened, men have to rationalise their position and negotiate, both within themselves and with their wives and families, about what to do. (White & Johnson, 2000, p.540)

What the above examples serve to illustrate is that – in the context of experiencing the symptoms of prostate cancer, testicular cancer and chest pain at least – constructions of hegemonic masculinity can and do have a deleterious influence on men's decision to seek and access medical help in a timely manner. Yet, these studies still leave the equivalent problem of homogeneity that is evident in those investigations employing a gender-role socialisation analytical framework. That is, do *all* men adhere to these hegemonic versions of masculinity and, if not, how do 'other' masculinities intersect with men's help-seeking decision-making? Chapple and colleagues (2004) state this as a caveat in the report of their study findings, noting that although fear of damaging masculine self-image had influenced their (white, heterosexual) male subjects' reluctance to admit the need for medical help when experiencing the symptoms of testicular cancer: 'it is important to remember that there are many masculinities, and that male "roles" will vary depending on class, age and ethnicity' (p.31).

This 'pluralizing' of masculinity – the recognition of multiple masculinities – has been a central tenet of the social constructionist gender framework. Connell's (2005) influential work contrasted the culturally authoritative, hegemonic pattern of masculinity with less powerful representations of gender practice. The framework emphasises that other masculinities coexist, or more precisely are produced at the same time as hegemonic masculinity. These include marginalised and subordinated masculinities: gender forms produced in exploited or oppressed groups such as gay men and men from an ethnic minority (Connell, 2005). Despite this complexity, masculinity has often been essentialised and reduced to a singular construct by men's health researchers – the stereotypical white, heterosexual, hegemonic man – and deployed in relation to the 'damaging' association between men's help-seeking behaviour and the social construction of masculinity (Gough, 2006). The aforementioned studies on men's help-seeking behaviour, both empirically and theoretically, predominantly embody a distinctly white, monolithic and ultimately digressive perspective of masculinity (Galdas et al., 2005; Oliffe et al., 2007), and accounts of help-seeking from wider groups of men are conspicuously absent.

## Masculinities, identity and help-seeking behaviour

Recognising these limitations and the resultant gap in the men's help-seeking literature, O'Brien and colleagues (2005) endeavoured to explore how men of different age, life stage and social background considered consulting for symptoms of ill-health in relation to their masculinity. Analysing data collected from focus groups with 50 men living in Scotland (including healthy men, and groups of men who had prostate cancer, heart disease, mental health problems and ME), the researchers reported a widespread reluctance to seeking medical help and attributed this to subjects' 'hegemonic stance on masculinity' that men should be strong and stoical in the face of ill-health. Mirroring the findings of the studies discussed earlier on men with testicular and prostate cancer, being seen to endure pain and be 'strong and silent' in the face of illness, especially with respect to mental health and emotional problems, was widely viewed as a key practice of masculinity by the male respondents. However, of particular interest in this study was the additional finding that seeking medical help was a behaviour *embraced* by some subjects when it was perceived as a means of preserving or restoring another more valued representation of masculinity. These exceptions in the data are noteworthy because they serve to highlight the complexity of how intersections of hegemonic masculinity and help-seeking might be 'lived out' among differing groups of men. One interpretation of this data put forward by the researchers is that men may perceive seeking medical help to be lower in a 'hierarchy of threats' to their masculinity in comparison to the damaging impact an illness could potentially have on their masculine roles. Accordingly, seeking medical help promptly may in fact be perceived by some men as a means of managing or preserving, not threatening, their masculine identity. To illustrate, O'Brien and colleagues (2005) cite several firefighters in their study who were noted to place great emphasis on seeking medical help promptly – even for trivial symptoms – because it allowed them to maintain an occupational role that provided access to a hypermasculine identity, i.e. a healthy firefighter. A number of other men talked of a similar 'trade-off', noting that they would much rather risk their masculine status by consulting for a sexual health problem than put it at greater jeopardy by not being able to have sex.

What is particularly striking about O'Brien et al.'s (2005) study overall is that, despite the researchers having explicitly set out to explore the how a 'multiplicity of masculinities' might be constructed by men of differing age, life stage and occupation, their investigation in fact revealed how men use differing resources (primarily relating to their occupation) to construct culturally dominant (hegemonic) masculine ideals rather than addressing the issue of whether aspects of men's identities interplay with the construction of *differing (non-dominant) masculinities* in the context of seeking medical help. More recent attempts to address this gap in the literature have yielded some of the most interesting insights into men's help-seeking behaviour to date.

In one such study, Robertson (2003) explored the gender-related health practices of gay men, disabled men and able-bodied heterosexual men, highlighting some distinct differences between the groups. Drawing specifically on particular aspects of their identity which were allied to (supposedly) feminine ideals, the gay men who were interviewed talked of positive health and help-seeking practices and, moreover, distanced themselves from a stoical, hegemonic 'straight' male stance toward the use of health services. Similarly, the disabled men in the study were noted to use their specific impairment as a means of justifying engaging in 'healthy' behaviour (Robertson, 2003). What is particularly valuable about Robertson's results is that they point toward aspects of men's identity – in this case sexuality and disability – that may influence whether they attend to their health problems in a timely manner (or choose to adhere to hegemonic masculine ideals of being strong, stoical and not showing weakness) as reflected by subjects' differing perceptions about when it is acceptable or justifiable for a man to seek medical help. In view of these findings he argues that the stereotyping of 'men' in general as not wanting to take responsibility for their health and of consistently delaying seeking help cannot be sustained. Findings from subsequent studies conducted by Emslie et al. (2006) and Galdas et al. (2007) have served to support his assertion and, moreover, have added a further layer of depth and complexity to theories on the interrelationship between masculinities and men's help-seeking behaviour.

Reporting on the findings of 16 interviews conducted with men diagnosed with depression, Emslie and colleagues (2006) have noted that men use differing resources to construct or resist hegemonic masculine ideals. Current prevailing constructionist theories of masculinity would suggest that depression is 'incompatible' with dominant masculine values since the hegemonic script requires men to be tough, self-reliant and unemotional, and depression is symbolically assimilated with emotional weakness, vulnerability and femininity in western culture (Warren, 1983; Connell, 2005; Emslie et al., 2006). Although the researchers identified evidence to support this (some depressed men were seen to draw on hegemonic values associated with suppressing emotion and suicidal thoughts) they also found that several subjects actively constructed a narrative based around 'difference' from hegemonic masculinity. These men explicitly reflected on different ways of being masculine which were outside hegemonic masculine discourses; emphasising attributes such as creativity, sensitivity and intelligence in the context of experiencing and undergoing treatment for depression. The significance of these results from a social constructionist viewpoint is that they build on the findings from Robertson's study by illustrating other (non-dominant) constructions of masculinity that can have *positive* effects on men's health behaviour, further highlighting the complex nature of masculinities and their interplay with men's health. Emslie et al.'s (2006) research illustrates that men will not always attempt to 'live up' to hegemonic masculine ideals, can and will seek help for emotional or mental health problems, and thus that the generalisation that men are 'strong and silent' in the face of illness may reflect a simplistic version of what is in fact a complex story.

This complexity has been illuminated further by research that has explored the potentially emasculating problem of impotence following prostate cancer and the experiences of South Asian men seeking help for chest pain. Men have been found to be willing to talk about their emotional and physical experiences relating to impotence, further putting into question 'the much cited stoicism' often cited as the dominant masculine construction stopping men from talking about, and seeking help for, their health problems (Oliffe, 2005, p.9). Similarly, Galdas and colleagues (2007) have found that South Asian men seeking help for cardiac chest pain in the UK did not perceive a need to adhere to dominant hegemonic forms of masculinity that embody the perception of men as naturally strong, resistant to disease and unresponsive to pain and physical distress. By contrast, most Indian and Pakistani men in this study emphasised seeking prompt medical help when experiencing chest pain to be *gender-appropriate behaviour* for a South Asian man, and refuted strongly that others (such as wives, friends and colleagues) would view them as weak or less 'manly' as a result. One participant in the study, for example, explained that he did not live like 'that' [the western hegemonic masculine stereotype]:

*Researcher*: Were you worried at all that it [your symptoms] might be something serious or something to do with your heart?

**Participant**: Never came into my mind.

*Researcher*: But you went to see your doctor anyway?

**Participant**: Yes, to find out what it was. As it was, we don't have any appointments like in the morning so I went straight in and I told them and I had to wait about 5 or 10 minutes.

*Researcher*: Some men tend to put off going to see the doctor . . . some talk about a macho type attitude to put up with pain, can you identify with that at all? Do you see what I mean? Like, they don't want to appear soft or weak to other people and things if they go to the doctor.

**Participant**: No, no, no, I don't live like that. I mean if you are not feeling well you got to go to doctor.

Other men in Galdas et al.'s (2007) study similarly talked of their decision to visit the doctor as being 'very basic' and 'logical' on realising that pain was not responding to analgesia. Correspondingly, a number of South Asian men noted that they had visited their GP frequently in the past, and had few inhibitions about seeking help from their doctor when they had experienced chest pain:

**Participant**: I've always gone to the doctors straight away when I think something is wrong, he will tell me . . . If I am poorly I go to the doctor, simple as that'

The Indian and Pakistani men's narratives in this study clearly indicated that seeking medical help promptly was perceived as normative and therefore behaviour that was not a threat to their masculine identity. One explanation for this, as argued by the researchers, is that despite living in a western culture, most South Asian men did not consider western hegemonic representations of masculinity to be – as current social constructionist gender frameworks assert (Kimmel, 1996; Courtenay, 2000; Connell, 2005) – the masculinity that 'sets the standards' for all other men in the context of medical help-seeking. As explored further in Chapter 9, this, and other similar work, points toward the enactment of masculinity and its implications for health as being inextricably tied to a multitude of biographic factors, including ethnic identity.

## Conclusion

Although this chapter has shown that it remains vital for health professionals, policy-makers and researchers to be mindful of the potentially deleterious influence of hegemonic masculine ideals that emphasise power, control and stoicism on some men's help-seeking behaviour, the discussion has illustrated that the simplistic notion of 'men' being consistently averse to seeking medical help in a timely manner is not wholly supported by the empirical evidence. What the analysis in this chapter has shown instead is that men's decisions to seek or delay seeking medical help involves a complex intersectionality of gender, identity and social context. Recent studies have highlighted that 'living up' to hegemonic masculine ideals may not always be central in men's perception of their identity in the context of their help-seeking related decision-making and interactions. Rather, there is growing evidence showing that at different times in their lives and in different settings, men may consider various factors as central or threatening to their masculine identity when experiencing the symptoms of ill-health. Ethnicity, sexuality, age or occupational role may be a dominant factor in men's gender representations at certain times and in certain settings, but not in others. As Hearn and Collinson (1994) have argued, multiple masculinities are likely to be constructed through the various positionings of the self and others with regard to interconnected social divisions of gender, ethnicity and class. Thus, inevitably, help-seeking and its relationship to masculine identity has a temporal element; it is both multiple and shifting, dependent on aspects of identity – such as being gay, disabled, a firefighter, or South Asian – which are likely to be prioritised over others in differing social contexts. In developing an empirical basis from which to inform interventions to effectively engage men with health services, it is important to understand the complexity of 'masculine' attributes and thus avoid universalising assumptions about hegemonic masculinity that propagates an essentialist discourse about the damaging affect of 'masculinity' on men's help-seeking behaviour.

## References

Addis, M.E. & Mahalik, J.R. (2003) Men, masculinity, and the contexts of help seeking. *American Psychologist*, **58**(1), 5–14.

Banks, I. (2001) No man's land: men, illness and the NHS. *British Medical Journal*, **323**, 1058–1060.

Bem, S.L. (1974) The measurement of psychological androgyny. *Journal of Consulting and Clinical Psychology*, **42**, 144–162.

Boehmer, U. & Clark, J.A. (2001) Communication about prostate cancer between men and their wives. *Journal of Family Practice*, **50**, 226–231.

Brannon, R. (1976) The male sex role: our culture's blueprint of manhood and what it's done for us lately. In: *The Forty-Nine Per Cent Majority* (eds D. David & R. Brannon), pp.1–45. Reading, MA: Addison-Wesley.

Broom, A. (2004) Prostate cancer and masculinity in Australian society: a case of stolen identity? *International Journal of Men's Health*, **3**(2), 73–91.

Chapple, A. & Ziebland, S. (2002) Prostate cancer: embodied experience and perceptions of masculinity. *Social Health and Illness*, **24**, 820–841.

Chapple, A., Ziebland, S. & McPherson, A. (2004) Qualitative study of men's perceptions of why treatment delays occur in the UK for those with testicular cancer. *British Journal of General Practice*, **53**, 25–32.

Connell, R.W. (2000) *The Men and the Boys*. St. Leonards, NSW, Australia: Allen & Unwin.

Connell, R.W. (2005) *Masculinities*. Cambridge: Polity Press.

Connell, R.W. & Messerschmidt, J.W. (2005) Hegemonic masculinity: rethinking the concept. *Gender and Society*, **19**(6), 829–859.

Cook, D.G., Morris, J.K., Walker, M. & Sharper, A.G. (1990) Consultation rates among middle-aged men in general practice over three years. *British Medical Journal*, **301**, 647–650.

Corney, R.H. (1990) Sex differences in general practice attendance and help seeking for minor illness. *Journal of Psychosomatic Research*, **34**, 525–534.

Courtenay, W.H. (2000) Constructions of masculinity and their influence on men's well-being: a theory of gender and health. *Social Science and Medicine*, **50**(10), 1385–1401.

Courtenay, W.H. (2002) Behavioural factors associated with disease, injury and death among men: evidence and implications for prevention. *International Journal of Men's Health*, **1**(3), 281–342.

Department of Health (2000) *Press Release: reference 2000/0187*. London: The Stationery Office.

Eisler, R.M. & Skidmore, J.R. (1987) Masculine gender role stress: scale development and component factors in the appraisal of stressful situations. *Behaviour Modification*, **11**(2), 123–136.

Emslie, C. (2005) Women, men and coronary heart disease: a review of the qualitative literature. *Journal of Advanced Nursing*, **51**(4), 382–395.

Emslie, C., Ridge, D., Ziebland, S. & Hunt, K. (2006) Men's accounts of depression: reconstructing or resisting hegemonic masculinity? *Social Science and Medicine*, **62**, 2246–2257.

Evans, J., Butler, L., Etowa, J., Crawley, I., Rayson, D. & Bell, D.G. (2005) Gendered and cultured relations: exploring African Nova Scotians' perceptions and experiences of breast and prostate cancer. *Research and Theory for Nursing Practice: An International Journal*, **19**(3), 257–273.

Galdas, P.M., Cheater, F.M. & Marshall, P. (2005) Men and health help-seeking behaviour: literature review. *Journal of Advanced Nursing*, **49**(6), 616–623.

Galdas, P.M., Cheater, F.M. & Marshall, P. (2007) What is the role of masculinity on white and South Asian men's decision to seek medical help for cardiac chest pain? *Journal of Health Services Research and Policy*, **12**(4), 223–229.

Gascoigne, P. & Whitear, B. (1999) Making sense of testicular cancer symptoms: a qualitative study of the way in which men sought help from the health care services. *European Journal of Oncology Nursing*, **3**(2), 62–69.

George, A. & Fleming, P. (2004) Factors affecting men's help-seeking in the early detection of prostate cancer: implications for health promotion. *Journal of Men's Health and Gender*, **1**(4), 345–352.

GISSI (1986) [Gruppo Italiano per lo Studio Della Streptochiniasi Nell'Infarto Miocardico] Effectiveness of intravenous thrombolytic treatment in acute myocardial infarction. *Lancet*, **1**, 397–401.

GISSI (1995) Avoidable Delay Group [Gruppo Italiano per lo Studio Della Streptochiniasi Nell'Infarto Miocardico] Epidemiology of avoidable delay in the care of patients with acute myocardial infarction. *Archives of Internal Medicine*, **155**, 1481–1488.

Good, G.E., Dell, D.M. & Mintz, L.B. (1989) The male role and gender role conflict: relations to help seeking in men. *Journal of Counseling Psychology*, **36**, 295–300.

Gough, B. (2006) Try to be healthy, but don't forgo your masculinity: deconstructing men's health discourse in the media. *Social Science and Medicine*, **63**, 2476–2488.

Gray, R.E., Fitch, M., Phillips, C.L. et al. (2000) To tell or not to tell: patterns of disclosure among men with prostate cancer. *Psychooncology*, **9**, 273–282.

Harrison, J. (1978) Warning: the male sex role may be dangerous to your health. *Journal of Social Issues*, **34**(1), 65–86.

Harrison, J., Chin, J. & Ficarrotto, T. (1989) Warning: masculinity may be dangerous to your health. In: *Men's Lives* (eds M.S. Kimmel & M.A. Messner), pp.296–309. New York: Macmillan.

Health Development Agency (2002) *Young Men's Health: What Works and Why?* London: Health Development Agency Publications.

Hearn, J. (1994) Research in men and masculinities: some sociological issues and possibilities. *Australia and New Zealand Journal of Sociology*, **30**, 47–70.

Hearn, J. & Collinson, D.L. (1994) Theorizing unities and difference between men and between masculinities. In: *Theorizing Masculinities* (eds H. Brod and M. Kaufman), pp.97–118. London: Sage Publications.

Helgeson, V.S. (1995) Masculinity, men's roles and CHD. In: *Men's Health and Illness: Gender, Power, and the Body* (eds D. Sabo & D.F. Gordon), pp.68–104. London: Sage Publications.

Hewitt, A.K., Kainth, A., Pattenden, J. et al. (2004) *Predictors of Delay in Seeking Medical Help in Patients with Suspected Heart Attack, and Interventions to Reduce Delay: A Systematic Review.* Centre for Reviews and Dissemination, University of York, **26**, 1–141.

Husaini, B.A., Moore, S.T. & Cain V.A. (1994) Psychiatric symptoms and help seeking behavior among the elderly: an analysis of racial and gender differences. *Journal of Gerontological Social Work*, **21**, 177–193.

ISIS-2 (1988) Second international study of infarct survival. Collaborative group randomised trial of intravenous streptokinase, oral aspirin, both, or neither in 17 187 cases of suspected acute myocardial infarction. *Lancet*, **2**, 349–360.

Kimmel, M.S. (1996) *Manhood in America.* New York: Free Press.

Lee, C. & Owens, R.G. (2002) *The Psychology of Men's Health.* Buckingham, UK: Open University Press.

Macintyre, S., Hunt, K. & Sweeting, H. (1996) Gender differences in health: are things really as simple as they seem? *Social Science and Medicine*, **42**(4), 617–624.

Mansfield, A.K., Addis, M.E. & Mahalik, J.R. (2003) 'Why won't he go to the doctor?' The psychology of men's help seeking. *International Journal of Men's Health*, **2**(2), 93–109.

Mansfield, A.K., Addis, M.E. & Courtenay, W.H. (2005) Measurement of men's help seeking: development and evaluation of the barriers to help seeking scale. *Psychology of Men and Masculinity*, **6**(2), 95–108.

Mason, O.J. & Strauss, K. (2004) Testicular cancer: passage through the help-seeking process for a cohort of UK men (part 1). *International Journal of Men's Health*, **3**(2), 93–110.

McCarthy, J. & Holliday, E.L. (2004) Help seeking and counseling within a traditional male gender role: an examination from a multicultural perspective. *Journal of Counseling and Development*, **82**, 25–30.

McKay, J.R., Rutherford, M.J., Cacciola, J.S. et al. (1996) Gender differences in the relapse experiences of cocaine patients. *Journal of Nervous and Mental Disease*, **184**, 616–622.

Mechanic, D. (1978) Sex, illness, illness behaviour and the use of health services. *Social Science and Medicine*, **12B**, 207–214.

Men's Health Forum (2004) *Getting it Sorted: A Policy Programme for Men's Health*. London: Men's Health Forum.

Mendoza, J. & Cummings, A.L. (2001) Help-seeking and male gender-role attitudes in male batterers. *Journal of Interpersonal Violence*, **16**(8), 833–840.

Möller-Leimkühler, A.M. (2002) Barriers to help seeking by men: a review of sociocultural and clinical literature with particular reference to depression. *Journal of Affective Disorders*, **71**, 1–9.

Moynihan, C. (1998) Theories in health care and research: theories of masculinity. *British Medical Journal*, **317**(7165), 1072–1075.

NHS Executive (1998) *National Survey of NHS Patients: General Practice*. London: The Stationery Office.

O'Brien, R., Hunt, C. & Hart, G. (2005) 'It's cavemen stuff, but that is to a certain extent how guys still operate': men's accounts of masculinity and help seeking. *Social Science and Medicine*, **61**(3), 503–516.

Oliffe, J.L. (2005) Constructions of masculinity following prostatectomy-induced impotence. *Social Science and Medicine*, **60**, 2249–2259.

Oliffe, J.L., Grewal, S., Bottorff, J.L. et al. (2007) Elderly South Asian Canadian immigrant men: confirming and disrupting dominant discourses about masculinity and men's health. *Family and Community Health*, **30**(3), 224–236.

Padesky, C.A. & Hammen, C.L. (1981) Sex differences in depressive symptom expression and help-seeking among college students. *Sex Roles*, **7**, 309–320.

Pleck, J. (1981) *The Myth of Masculinity*. Cambridge, MA: MIT Press.

Pleck, J.H., Sonenstein, F.L. & Ku, L.C. (1994) Problem behaviours and masculinity ideology in adolescent males. In: *Adolescent Problem Behaviours: Issues and Research* (eds R.D. Ketterlinus & M.E. Lamb), pp.165–186. Hillsdale, NJ: Lawrence Erlbaum.

Robertson, S. (2003) Men managing health. *Men's Health Journal*, **2**(4), 111–113.

Sabo, D. & Gordon, D.F. (1995) Rethinking men's health and illness. In: *Men's Health and Illness: Gender, Power, and the Body* (eds D. Sabo & D.F. Gordon), pp.1–21. London: Sage Publications.

Saltonstall, R. (1993) Healthy bodies, social bodies: men's and women's concepts and practices of health in everyday life. *Social Science and Medicine*, **36**(1), 7–14.

Sharpe, S. & Arnold, S. (1998) Men, lifestyle and health: a study of health beliefs and practices. Unpublished Report on Project for ESRC (no R000221950).

Smith, J.A., Braunack-Mayer, A. & Wittert, G. (2006) What do we know about men's help-seeking and health service use? *Medical Journal of Australia*, **184**(2), 81–83.

Smith, L.K., Pope, C. & Botha, J.L. (2005) Patients' help-seeking experiences and delay in cancer presentation: a qualitative synthesis. *Lancet*, **366**, 825–831.

Spence, J.T., Helmreich, R.L. & Stapp, J. (1974) The personal attributes questionnaire: a measure of sex-role stereotypes and masculinity and femininity. *JSAS Catalogue of Selected Documents in Psychology*, **4**, 127.

Thom, B. (1986) Sex differences in help-seeking for alcohol problems: 1. Barriers to help-seeking. *British Journal of Addiction*, **81**, 777–788.

Tudiver, T. & Talbot, Y. (1999) Why don't men seek help? Family physicians' perspectives on help-seeking behavior in men. *Journal of Family Practice*, **48**(1), 47–52.

UKHAS (1998) (United Kingdom Heart Study) Collaborative Group. Effect of time from onset to coming under care on fatality of patients with acute myocardial infarction: effect of resuscitation and thrombolytic therapy. *Heart*, **80**, 121–126.

Waldron, I. (1976) Why do women live longer than men? *Social Science and Medicine*, **10**, 349–362.

Warren, L. (1983) Male intolerance of depression: a review with implications for psychotherapy. *Clinical Psychology Review*, **3**(2), 147–156.

Weissman, M.M. & Klerman, G.L. (1977) Sex differences and the epidemiology of depression. *Archives of General Psychiatry*, **34**, 98–111.

White, A.K. (2000) Men making sense of their chest pain. PhD Thesis, University of Manchester, UK.

White, A.K. (2001) Report on the scoping study on men's health. Unpublished Research Report. Leeds Metropolitan University/HMSO, UK.

White, A.K. & Johnson, M. (2000) Men making sense of their chest pain – niggles, doubts and denials. *Journal of Clinical Nursing*, **9**(4), 534–541.

White, A.K., Fawkner, H.J. & Holmes, M. (2006) Is there a case for differential treatment of young men and women? *Medical Journal of Australia*, **185**(5), 454–455.

# Chapter 4

# GENDER AND PSYCHOSOCIAL ADAPTATION AFTER A CORONARY EVENT: A RELATIONAL ANALYSIS

Don Sabo and Julia Hall

## Introduction

Gender scholars have mainly focused on health and illness *within* each sex rather than *between* the sexes. In contrast, relational theories of gender and health recognise that men's and women's health processes and outcomes are intricately interconnected (Sabo, 1999; Schofield et al., 2000). As Schofield et al. (2000, p.251) stated, 'A gender relations approach is one that proposes that men's and women's interactions with each other, and the circumstances under which they interact, contribute significantly to health opportunities and constraints.' Similarly, Payne (2006) discusses the complex biological, cultural, social and economic processes that influence the respective health of men and women, but she also traces how the intersections between men's and women's roles within varying institutional contexts and power relationships can shape each gender's diagnosis and treatment, access to and utilisation of healthcare, and psychosocial adaptation to illness and recovery. Stated another way, men's and women's health unfold within relationships that are situated in various institutional contexts or what Connell (1987) refers to as 'gender regimes', and it is through these relational processes that psychosocial adaptation to coronary heart disease is given shape and direction.

The qualitative study explored here focuses on the relational aspects of men's and women's psychosocial reactions and adjustments after a coronary event. Coronary heart disease (CHD) is the single leading cause of mortality in the United States and 13.2 million people in the current population have a history of heart attack, angina pectoris (chest pains), or both. Each year an estimated 1.2 million people will have a new or recurrent coronary event (Thom et al., 2006). The aetiology and health outcomes associated with CHD are influenced by the social and economic relations of gender, class, race and sexuality. For example, mortality due to CHD among specific groups of women and men recently declined due to improved interventions, nutrition and exercise education, and an increased attention to health promotion. This is not the case, however, for marginalised women and men, who may lack adequate health insurance, have high stress, and may not have the time, ability, or cultural propensity to focus on health maintenance education and prevention (Edwards et al., 2005). As CHD impacts through communities, social class and race/ethnicity are revealed to be large predictors in the morbidity and mortality rates for those grappling with this condition. Poor and working-class men were less able to reconstruct their post-coronary gender identities and lifestyles after a coronary event than their more affluent counterparts (Sabo et al., 2006).

Numerous gender differences in coronary care and outcomes have been documented. Biomedical research after World War II focused mainly on men, as women were not selected as research subjects. Because cardiac diagnostic tests, medications and surgical procedures were researched and developed using mainly males as subjects, many biological, anatomical and physiological differences between women and men were discounted (Legato, 2000). Until recently, there was little recognition of different coronary symptoms between the sexes; for example, while men typically experience left arm and chest pain, dizziness and shortness of breath, women often exhibit back, abdomen and throat pain (Edwards et al., 2005). Compared to men, women are less likely to be recommended, after initial clinical presentation, for angioplasty and angiograms. After treatment, fewer women than men are referred to cardiac rehabilitation (McSweeney & Coon, 2004) and, if they enrol, women are reported to be less apt than men to complete the cycles of cardiac rehabilitation (Halm et al., 1999). Among working women, attrition rates are linked to lower wage and inadequate health benefits compared to men. Key factors are the pressures of managing family and work, as well as feelings of guilt when taking time away from caregiving (McSweeney & Coon, 2004). Despite the fact that women's risk of heart attack dramatically increases after menopause, older women, who may be widowed or divorced, may forgo cardiac rehabilitation due to financial constraints, transportation barriers and lack of spousal support (Benz-Scott et al., 2002; Farley et al., 2003; McSweeney & Coon, 2004; Jackson et al., 2005; Peddicord, 2005).

While many women de-prioritise their health needs, many also do not understand the key warning signs of CHD, and encounter clinical practices in coronary care that are geared primarily toward males. Findings show that men often deny symptoms of illness, ignore preventive health information, avoid seeking help and under-utilise healthcare services (Addis & Mahalik, 2003; Evans et al., 2005). Men engage in fewer health-promoting behaviours than women (Courtenay, 2000, 2002) and often turn to so-called denial or distraction to avoid personal responsibility for their health (Stanton & Courtenay, 2003). The 'demands of the male role', stress and symptom denial have been tied to men's risk of coronary heart disease (Harrison et al., 1992; Sabo, 2005).

In addition to the above gender influences, variations in men's and women's health are shaped within historical and social contexts of race, ethnicity, and economic inequalities (Zierler & Krieger, 1997). People of colour in the US, for example, disproportionately face economic disadvantages, racism, unemployment and under-utilisation of healthcare. Poverty and lower educational attainment also mitigate against the adoption of preventive health behaviours and adaptation to chronic illness (Sabo, 2005). While the bulk of epidemiological research examines the aetiology and prevalence of CHD among racial and ethnic minorities and economically disadvantaged groups, there is a paucity of research focusing on the psychosocial aspects of treatment and recovery. In a previous qualitative study of a diverse sample of men recovering from a coronary incident, we found their long-term efforts to redefine their identities and lifestyles in more healthful directions were influenced by complex interplays between social class and race/ethnicity (Sabo et al., 2006). The least favourable preventive outcomes occurred when the potential for racial and ethnic marginalisation was melded with lower socioeconomic status. In contrast, men from higher socioeconomic strata, regardless of colour, enjoyed a greater range of options for redefining their identities and lifestyles in healthful ways.

From the outset, the current exploratory study took a general relational approach to describing and examining how the interfaces between men's and women's lives influence each gender's psychosocial adaptation during treatment and recovery from a coronary event. The key research questions included:

(1) What are the patterns of men's and women's psychosocial reactions and adjustments after a coronary event and how are these patterns similar or different?
(2) How do gender relations influence women's and men's experiences and outcomes with regard to caregiving, care-receiving and extended recovery?
(3) To what extent are these gendered health processes and outcomes influenced by the interplay among social class and race/ethnicity?

In the conclusion, we examine the notion of 'gendered health synergies' (Sabo, 1999) as related to the experiences of the men and women interviewed here.

## Method

This analysis is based on semi-structured, open-ended interviews with the intent to describe and analyse women's and men's psychosocial adjustments to diagnosis, treatment and recovery following a coronary event. The purposive sample consisted of 40 economically and culturally diverse women and men, 45 to 70 years old, who had experienced a coronary event that required some type of hospitalisation, such as angioplasty, valve replacement or bypass surgery. In all but one case, only women and men who experienced a coronary event 6 to 36 months prior to interviewing were selected. Pseudonyms are used throughout this chapter when referring to individual participants.

Four pilot interviews were carried out prior to the current study in order to develop an interview guide that used a basic life history approach (Bogdan & Biklen, 2006) to trace women's and men's lives before the actual coronary event, their experiences during diagnosis and treatment, and during the period of protracted recovery. The main lines of inquiry included perceptions of the causes of their condition, how they defined and felt about CHD, their health beliefs and practices prior to diagnosis and treatment, and their experiences during treatment and recovery. Special focus was placed on the long-term recovery phase and the extent to which they had changed their daily routines, physical activity, nutritional practices, other health behaviours and overall personal identity. Throughout the interviews, we evoked reflection and conversation about whom the participants relied on for knowledge and care, how CHD might have changed their body concepts, and the ways they saw themselves as women and men.

As white male and female college professors and researchers, we were mindful of the dangers of speaking for others, and were aware that individual experiences with heart disease are mediated by family and community history. Because one objective was to recruit those who are often excluded from health research due to cultural and/or economic marginalisation, the sample included African American, Puerto Rican, Native American and white participants. We worked with a Spanish-speaking Latina colleague to interview Puerto Rican women and men and the tapes were transcribed into English. A Native American professor likewise interviewed First Nations participants. We discussed interpretations at the data analysis stage with these individuals. We located participants using our own personal networks and the snowball effect, which undoubtedly impacted the sample (Bogdan & Biklen, 2006).

Throughout this research, considering the social class and race/ethnicity of participants, we used various terms with which they self-identify and/or made inferences based on their occupation and life histories. We understood categories such as 'poor', 'working class', 'middle class' and 'upper middle class' as fluid boundaries, made even more so in an unstable economy. Weis (2004) argues, though, that while material locations such as 'working class' are under massive assault in the present economy, the discursive cultural and behavioural elements of these factions still hold familiar meanings. For the purposes of this work, 'poor/low income' refers to those who rely on social services; 'working class' refers to those in the subordinate primary labour market; 'middle class' refers to those in the primary labour market; and 'upper middle class' refers to those who work in the supervisory or intellectual realm of the primary labour market (Weis, 2004; Anyon, 2005).

The data analysis followed a grounded theory approach that used an inductive-deductive process for learning about and explaining reality (Glaser & Strauss, 1967; Glaser, 1978; Watson, 2000). We partly saw ourselves as storytellers; that is, researchers who set out to compile narratives of those we encountered. The first task was to describe, and later, amid a growing reservoir of texts and insights, to identify themes and to ascribe meanings to participants' experiences.

## Living in denial

All 21 men interviewed denied their risk for heart disease during the years prior to diagnosis and treatment. This denial is all the more telling, considering that the males described many instances of heart disease within their family histories, and current lives full of unhealthy diets, high levels of stress and, in a few cases, smoking and drug usage. Ironically, denial among these males was based on the very fact they were holding down high-pressure jobs, or involved in physical activity on a daily basis; some were running marathons and participating in extreme sports and adventure travel or had lived through military combat, thus proving their 'toughness'. The seamless denial of CHD among the male participants emerged out of a meaning-making process based on a belief system in which the masculine body is invincible.

The denial of risk among the men took many forms. Several men reported being too busy or engaged in work to fret about heart disease. Rick, a white working-class maintenance worker, said he never paid any attention to his health because he 'usually worked six days a week, anywhere from 8 to 12, 13, 14 hours a day'. Bradley, an upper middle-class African American retiree, described how, despite his mother dying of a heart attack and three of his five sisters being diagnosed with heart disease, he 'never thought me'. Other men assumed that as long as they remained physically active, that is, going back and forth to work, exercising, travelling, the odds were heart disease would pass them by. Claude, a white college professor and distance runner whose father had died from heart disease at age 47, explained, 'I never thought of me having heart disease. If you can run marathons, your heart must be okay.' Lance, an upper middle-class African American business owner, whose father died after his third heart attack, said proudly, 'I was Mr Fitness . . . I have always been physically fit.'

In addition to taking refuge from the threat of CHD through the enactment of male roles such as the hard worker, fitness buff or athlete, masculinity also threaded through participants' personal identities and body concepts. Jack, a retired white middle-class police officer and Vietnam veteran, reflected on how he participated in the risk-laden male police subculture. 'You smoke and eat shit food and drink,' he recalled, 'you do everything you can to try and commit suicide. Not consciously, but under the (culture).' He considered himself a strong and powerful man who 'survived Vietnam' and who once 'hiked to the bottom of the Grand Canyon and slept in a tent'. His masculine self-image helped mask his vulnerability to heart disease. Several men simply rationalised their risk away. For example, in thinking about the extent of obesity among his relatives, Ricardo, a working-class Puerto Rican male reflected:

*Heart problems run in my family. My dad died of a heart attack and my grandfather did not die of a heart attack, but he did have heart problems. No one really talked about it, so I don't know the names of the conditions my family members had. I always just thought that I would never have any medical problems.*

When the risk for CHD became conscious, it was whisked away.

In reflecting upon their lives before their coronary event, of the 13 women interviewed, all but one evidenced deep strains of denial that heart disease would affect them, despite the fact that coronary conditions plagued their families. The lone female who did expect to have coronary difficulty, a low-income Native American named Sandy, was born with a heart condition that has resulted in ongoing hospitalisation and near-death experiences her entire life. Similar to the men, given the prevalence of males *and* females in past generations in their lives who encountered heart disease, it is startling how repeatedly, the majority thought 'it would never happen to me'. Gladys, a middle-class African American, saw her father battle heart disease, but never thought she would be at risk, even though she smokes, admits to a high cholesterol diet and has a high stress job as a social worker. Barbara, a middle-class African American, stated that she did not feel she was at risk, even though her grandmother and daughter had heart problems. Denial for these women is based on the belief they are 'immune' to heart disease due to their biological gender, the fact they do not have time to be sick due to their 'caretaker' role, and for some, the 'protection' they receive through deep spiritual beliefs.

Most of the women constructed their central identity as 'caretaker', and it was enacted daily in the forms of wife, partner, mother and daughter. The identity construction of the steadfast caretaker also required that one be a 'survivor'. Olga, a low-income Puerto Rican, who lived through financial struggle, an unstable childhood, an abusive marriage, divorce, and unhealthy food patterns, said she 'knew it [heart disease] was in the family, but never thought it would affect me. I was a strong woman who had been affected by many things but survived.' She described how she regularly gave blood and filled out her organ donor card, and how she always saw herself as helping others. Katie, an upper middle-class white educator and athlete, explains how her heart attack 'came out of left field', especially since she is a cancer survivor and is physically fit. For the most part, these women see their success as caretakers as predicated on the fact that, in many ways, they are all survivors.

Almost all the women also said they did not expect to become a CHD statistic because they thought it was a 'man's disease'. Especially once in their late 20s, 30s, 40s and beyond, they were focused on avoiding, or at least learning about, female-specific health conditions such as breast and cervical cancer and, to them, heart disease was not part of this 'package'. Susan, a white, working-class woman with a history of heart problems since young adulthood, talked about how her father, grandmother and grandfather died young from heart disease, yet somehow she did not feel she was at risk. She said simply, 'I figured I was a woman and it would not affect me.' Arlene said in the past she thought of CHD as a man's disease: 'You would hear about men who had a sudden heart attack and died.' Despite her mother having a heart attack, and her own habit of smoking and eating on the run, she never thought it would enter into her orbit. Martha, a working-class Puerto Rican, said she 'always thought heart problems were a male disease. I always thought men died of heart attacks.'

Another unique facet of denial among 5 out of 13 women was a belief that the coronary event was somehow a spiritual test. Susan explained how she wrestled to accept her diagnosis: 'it was part of God's plan and the way he wanted to work in my life . . . he wants you to trust him because he loves you.' Barbara, who is married to a minister and lost a daughter to cancer years ago, feels there is a spiritual plan in her life, with heart disease playing its part. Gladys gained strength when her husband and children prayed over her while waking up from surgery. She leaves crucial events like this 'in the Lord's hands', and prayed with her pastor and a good friend on the telephone the night before her surgery. Olga believed 'God works in mysterious ways. There is a reason for my illness to come into my life at the time it did. I do not have the answer for this but God knows.' Jane, a low-income white female, also described how she would take comfort by praying to God for help and answers to her problems.

## Coping with diagnosis, treatment and recovery

On diagnosis, and during initial treatment and recovery, very different coping mechanisms appeared across gender lines. The men for the most part relied heavily on their wives and partners for decision-making, emotional support and caregiving. For this small but intense span of time, the men relinquished their masculine exteriors and completely gave in to the nurturing care of the women in their lives. This phase is characterised by sheer emotion – fear, anxiety, anger, depression, guilt and a sudden feeling of being fully dismantled by their health crisis. As time went on, during protracted recovery, a stronger sense of self and a clearer future came to light. As part of piecing their lives back together, some men reverted to the previously established, more traditional role of the dominant male, while others continued to stay more in touch with their emotions and to be more open and dependent on their partners.

For example, after initially resisting acceptance of his heart condition, Sam, a white middle-class carpenter and home builder who prides himself on the physicality of his work, finally gave into his diagnosis and turned over his care to his wife. As a nurse, his wife interfaced with doctors and hospital staff, and when Sam went home she tended to his needs while he recuperated. During his initial diagnosis and recovery, he became almost childlike, completely relying on his wife for caregiving and nurturance. Today, now several years later, gender relations have returned to 'normal' and he has resumed work, but not as compulsively as he worked before the heart attack. Bradley, a high-level, go-getter executive, completely gave himself over to his wife's care during diagnosis and treatment. He became so fully dependent on her presence that even today he needs her by his side nearly all the time.

In comparison, the women in the study who had spouses or partners only minimally turned to the men in their lives for emotional support and care during the initial crisis and treatment period, and also during long-term recuperation. For the females, the sheer terror of the immediate diagnosis, in almost every case, was paralleled by the reactionary urge to 'protect' their families from experiencing this fear. The women made a conscious decision to spare their spouse/partner from the stress of the situation. They put up brave fronts, shielded husbands and children from upsetting information and even, at times, requested that their partners stay home instead of sit at their bedside in the hospital and intensive care unit (ICU). These females all spoke about how they worried about their families, and even felt guilty for putting them through this crisis. The women, despite being terrified about their chances of survival at this crucial juncture, went into full 'nurture and protect' mode when it came to their families.

Support for the women, both single and partnered, during initial crisis and recovery, was drawn from sources of mostly female networks. Joan, a white upper middle-class landscape business owner, said she received strength from a tight circle of female friends, in order that her husband could have time and space to come to grips with her open-heart surgery. Susan explained that in order to 'shield' her husband she leaned on a friend. Barbara talked about how she felt better leaning on women from her church instead of her husband, daughters and parents, because she could not stand to see them so upset over her condition. Rosie, a lower middle-class white woman, said she depended more on her daughters than her husband, because although he was wonderfully supportive she wanted to protect him, and felt eventually he would want her to toughen up. Gladys described how she used her sense of independence and deep faith in God to ensure that she could sustain her husband and children during the ordeal. Each of these women, including those who did not have a partner, also described how during this traumatic time they drew on unknown reserves of inner strength, constructing and tapping into the 'survivor within'.

## Reconstructing gender identity during extended recovery

For several of the men and women in this study, it was only by sidestepping the more traditional male and female family patterns that they were able to construct healthier choices and lifestyles. Traditional relational dynamics carry heavy cultural burdens, such as the subjectivity of male-as-breadwinner and female-as-caretaker. As a whole, the male and female participants exhibited a range of gender identity reconstruction arrangements during protracted recovery.

## Findings among men

Throughout their lives, most had come to view a wide array of masculine identities and traits. As younger men, most had come to view their bodies as invulnerable to pain or illness. To an extent, toughness was equated to masculinity. Yet when hit by the diagnosis and initial treatment and recovery, they were completely knocked off their feet, shattered, needy and dependent on their partners. In addition to physical healing, their long road to recovery also involved rethinking and reformulating their sense of masculine identity. Some embraced and tried to understand the vulnerabilities, dependencies and raw emotions they experienced. They attempted to stay in touch with these relatively new sides of themselves, to forge deeper bonds with their partners and to explore the need to express and receive intimacy.

During the extended recovery phase, the men resolved to repair their bodies, enact new behaviours, and to live as long as they could in good health. Despite these intentions, their narratives revealed three types of long-term adaptation, which to a large extent represent clusters characterised by the social class standing and race of participants. The lower-income men made an initial effort to change their body image and masculine identity, but due to their inability to work or find a job, their lack of insurance and general financial stress, they ultimately drifted back to the same self-image, behaviours and denial that existed before the onset of CHD. The middle-income men reported doing a great deal of soul-searching during recovery. They initially re-examined their relationships with family, changed their diets, lost weight and increased their levels of physical activity. Across months and years, however, they found themselves slipping in and out of old habits. They cycled between weight loss and weight gain, returned to unhealthy 'family comfort foods', resumed smoking, pushed work and exercise to stressful levels, and only occasionally monitored information on CHD.

Finally, the upper middle-class males seemed particularly able to modify and reconstruct their gender identities. Some reported getting emotionally closer to their wives or children. One who felt more 'feminine' and caring said he now sought out friends with illnesses and visited them in the hospital or at home. They also talked about treating their bodies in less 'manly' ways; that is, not pushing themselves to the limit but being more oriented to self-care. Part of the flexibility to rethink and reshape the meanings surrounding masculinity in their lives and identities was facilitated by greater educational attainment, solid financial resources, premium medical insurance, personal contacts with health professionals, and the time and ability to use technology to access health information. Our analysis revealed that they not only succeeded in changing their identities and behaviours along preventive lines during the period of extended recovery, but they also maintained these changes over time. Many of these changes involved reconstructing identity outside traits associated with conventional masculinity production. For example, they remained in touch with their emotions around CHD, stayed attuned to their bodies, kept up with preventive health information and medical follow-ups, and nurtured closeness to partners, family and friends.

Among the lower-income men, Rick, Ricardo and Felix struggled to find direction in their recovery, and despite initial earnestness and some changes, they devolved into their old habits. For instance, because of the severity of his coronary condition and recovery, Rick was not able to stay with his job. He and his wife moved into the basement of their daughter's house, and his wife now has a part-time minimum wage job with no health insurance. The purchase of healthcare coverage puts a huge financial burden on his family. Although he lost some weight, he did not adopt a healthy diet or physical activity regime, and his cigarette addiction came back to haunt him.

After an initial push to change their lifestyles, several mostly middle-income men adopted a middle-of-the-road stance. A few upper middle-class men are also part of this subgroup. These men retained some pre-coronary risk behaviours and attitudes but developed preventive strategies as well. Stan, who is white and middle class, made many changes in terms of physical activity, but is not consistent in terms of nutrition. While Sam radically restructured his diet, increased his level of physical activity and lost 40 pounds, he continued to take on stressful home construction jobs. He also decided that he no longer needs to go to the doctor, as he now knows what he needs 'to treat himself'. In terms of diet, Claude also made some adjustments such a cutting down on red meat and chicken wings, but he re-adopted the same pre-coronary premise that operated before his heart surgery (i.e. being a runner means minimal risk for heart disease). While white, upper middle-class Jake made major adjustments in his life in terms of meditation and becoming educated on his condition, he spent half the year on the road in his high-pressure sales job, and has not significantly changed his diet or level of physical activity. These men continue to struggle to make behavioural and identity changes, but have not completely reverted to their old ways.

A third cluster of narratives was men who radically transformed their lives, bodies and identities in profound ways and, furthermore, maintained the healthful metamorphosis. Upper middle-class African American Jasper drastically altered his diet, exercise and outlook. He now exclusively eats oatmeal for breakfast and a low-fat, mostly vegetarian diet for lunch and dinner. He exercises every morning for an hour. He is upbeat about the future, wants to be around to see his great grandchildren, and is in close contact with the healthcare system. White, upper middle-class Gary rises every day at 3:30 a.m. to work out. He also participates in a cardiac support group, and through this organisation visits patients in the hospital who are going through open-heart surgery. He said, 'I call this give-back time, right now it's my time to give back.' Bradley 'got closer' to his wife and they implemented a healthy lifestyle together full of exercise, proper nutrition and stress-reducing activities. By getting in touch with their emotions, these men created spaces outside established male gender configurations, which worked to support their healthy lifestyle.

The men's long-term recovery and efforts to reinvent themselves in terms of diet, exercise, relationships and general good health entailed self-evaluation and personal changes influenced by family and community support, access to heathcare and information, the ability to speak English, and financial resources. But each man's recovery was also informed by gender expectations and demands. The men's tendencies and capacity for denial of risk and symptoms for CHD were suffused by the cultural delusion that 'real men' are hard and invulnerable, that they endure pain silently, control their own lives and avoid dependency. The gendered workings for denial were at once somatic, psychological and cultural. In other words, if threatened by a fear of illness or if an odd pain in their chest reached consciousness or stirred anxiety, the awareness was suppressed and they moved on with their day's work, or they took refuge in the presumption that they were invulnerable and tough enough to endure. Like athletes enjoined by competition, they convinced themselves not consciously to care about the risk. The few men who were able to reconstruct a sense of self outside the margins of traditional masculinity fared the best in terms of long-term recovery.

**Findings among women**

The women's efforts to redefine themselves during recovery were deeply moored within the caretaker and protector identity in the forms of wife, partner, mother, daughter or employee. For example, while in the hospital, many women talked about struggling to be 'strong' for their husband and children so they could lean on them during the ordeal. In fact, many women never relinquished the caretaker identity in the first place, even in the ICU and during the most acute stages of diagnosis and treatment. They talked about how they tapped into their 'inner strength' in order to reconstruct their previous caretaker role as quickly as possible. For most of the women, caretaking was either consciously or unconsciously equated with survival. The 'survivor' narrative, based on the premise that what does not kill you makes you stronger, played throughout the life histories of these female participants and appears to be motivated by the belief that there is no time for self-pity, because others require your physical and emotional energy. Taking their biographies together, the women have indeed been strong and they have survived a great deal including financial struggle, physical and verbal abuse, childbirth, the death of grown children, divorce, the death of a spouse, other catastrophic health problems, institutional racism and sexism, lack of health insurance or under-insurance, and low self-image. To a certain extent social class, as intersected by race and ethnicity, mediated their ability to more reasonably enact and sustain the caretaking identity in ways that also afford long-term health changes for themselves. From the sample, it was only the women who constructed lives on the borders of accepted female family patterns who were able to sustain the best health.

Similar to the men, the women also displayed a range of gender identity reconstruction dynamics. Sandy alone had difficulty reconstructing the caretaker identity after her coronary event, which dovetailed with a period of extreme chaos. Heart attacks, strokes and open-heart surgery had ripped through her life, leaving her too ill to work and subsisting on social services. At the same time her teenage son was killed in an automobile accident, she was going through an ugly divorce, and prior to that had lost her brother to suicide. After losing her family, home and any remaining financial resources, Sandy had difficulty finding direction during extended recovery. She now survives day-to-day, and has not changed her diet or exercise patterns since the coronary event. She does not seem to understand the medical aspects of her condition, and reports that she sporadically sees a changing array of doctors at her health clinic. Still, she finds great meaning in volunteering once or twice a week at the local bingo hall. Her ability to help others and 'caretake' in this way, according to her sentiment, is tremendously meaningful to her.

It was through reconstructing the 'caretaker' identity that a large cluster of women attempted to make changes in their lives immediately after their coronary event. This group contained a mix of lower- and middle-income females. Their efforts to revise and renew themselves, however, met a variety of obstacles that compromised the staying power of their subjective transformation. While in the hospital, Gladys 'really did not lean on anybody' in an attempt to spare her family from the details of her pacemaker surgery, and she made plans to change her diet, exercise and stress levels. During extended recovery, she went back to work, but eventually resumed smoking and her previous high-fat diet. The pressures of being the sole supporter of her family, working in a stressful environment, and her son's recent legal trouble, potentially triggered the return of these old behaviours. Still, Gladys reads up on health issues, particularly articles related to African American women, and uses this knowledge to make choices about which doctors she continues to see. As a result, she has a strong group of healthcare providers in whom she trusts.

Susan still talked about how she wants to make changes in terms of diet and health, and then scolds herself for not following through. She said she did not go to rehabilitation after her open heart surgery because she did not have adequate health insurance. While she did go to a check-up one year after surgery, faced with a 20-dollar fee and living on a tight budget, she decided to cut out medical appointments to save money because there is 'not a lot to go around with two young children' and, she added, 'I don't want to hear there are any more issues.' Similarly, Jane's recovery was seriously limited by financial struggles, lack of health insurance, compounding medical problems, and the absence of someone to care for her. Despite these deficits, she contacted a free cardiac support group she found in the telephone book, and is a regular member. She finds significant comfort in belonging to this organisation. Even though Jane had long had her daughter and granddaughter living with her, she did not talk about her health crisis and issues with them, in order to spare them anxiety. Having also survived breast cancer and a double mastectomy, Jane felt isolated, lonely and financially vulnerable, and yet she continued primarily to define herself as a protector of her daughter and granddaughter, as they also are plagued by financial and personal issues.

A disturbing subtext emerged among this cluster of women who initially planned on making healthy adjustments in their lives but saw the changes fall by the wayside. Some of these women could not move forward completely because of lifetime insecurities surrounding body image and weight. These women were confronted by the fact that the coronary event meant, in a sense, that their bodies had failed them or, more circuitously, that they had failed their bodies. During recovery, they were forced to assess and critique former diet and exercise patterns, and this preoccupation seemed to push them back into decade-old concerns about body esteem and culturally inscribed messages about feminine beauty and self-worth.

Out of the 13 women, when asked about diet and exercise, seven steered the conversation to talk about body dissatisfaction. Susan reported that she always 'feels heavy' and was ridiculed by her family as a child. She looks at images of models in magazines and 'never feels good or adequate enough'. She described herself as 'still overweight' today, although to the outside observer she appears to be a healthy size. She felt 'inadequate going to the doctor and getting on the scale because I am not the perfect body type'. She also disclosed that for the doctor appointments leading up to her surgery, she planned her visits so she had time to lose weight before each session.

Two women described decades of negative eating behaviours which continue to this day. Barbara said while growing up 'she hated food' and even 'hated the feel of food' in her mouth. Her father would actually try to feed her with a teaspoon. After entering adulthood, marriage, and the birth of her three daughters, she still struggled with her weight. She was once hospitalised for weighing only 79 pounds, and stands at 5 feet 4 inches. Today, she eats breakfast and either lunch or dinner, and rides her exercise bike 50 miles a day. Similarly, Rosie admitted to battling several 'food phobias' concerning mayonnaise, salad dressings, vinegar and mustard, and she explained, 'I always felt I was fat.' Both of these women said they are still fixated on food and weight. We can only speculate about the extent that these body esteem issues were tied to earlier psychosocial efforts to attain 'feminine' body ideals within the dominant culture. The 'disconnect' with one's own body, as evidenced by the females in this subset, is likely a response, in part, to burdensome cultural messages about the production of femininity. These women expressed anger at themselves for what they viewed as continuing to put their families in jeopardy through their health crises. Not feeling thin and attractive enough, not good enough as a wife and caregiver, and continuously putting their own needs aside, they extend self-anger here through detachment from self, and seemingly punish themselves by 'controlling' their bodies.

Many of the women discussed conflicts about food in addition to what they themselves consume. Several mothers felt guilty for exposing their children to what they now perceived as poor nutrition. Susan said remorse-fully, 'I did not really lay down a good foundation when the kids were younger . . . I think all four of us are overweight.' Olga also lamented,

*It actually hurts me to think I was teaching my kids to cook so unhealthy. I would tell them lard was better to cook with because it would make*

*the rice or fried foods taste better . . . That's my job as a mother and I failed.*

Middle-class Native American Rita pointed to larger social forces at play, as she said, 'Europeans gave Native people two forms of self-destruction, rum and lard.' She described this as a process of victimisation, resulting in dietary abuses and excesses, and high rates of diabetes and heart disease that were crushing the community. Due to her new knowledge, she expressed anger for 'falling into the trap' of a poor diet.

Compounding a lifetime of low body image issues, several women described how, due to surgical scars, they feel even less physically desirable. Susan was concerned her husband would find her 8-inch chest scar unappealing, as she said that especially now, she is 'not a perfect image of what a body should look like'. Rosie explained how it pained her to look at herself in the mirror and see the scar, and she talked about making great strides in trying to accept this change. Sandy said she has been embarrassed about her boyfriend seeing her body. She is 'disgusted with her body and the way she looks', and has great trouble accepting a compliment about her appearance from anyone. Only one woman in this cluster, a working-class Puerto Rican named Pierrette, said she felt good about her body and sense of femininity. The rest were bogged down to varying degrees in culturally inscribed feelings of guilt and inadequacy.

While men's tendencies to deny the warning signs of CHD emerge from the cultural aberration that real men are tough, work through pain and shun dependency, the women's denial is grounded in taking care of others and setting their own needs aside. Already plagued with culturally based feelings of failure, these females see their scars as another major assault on their sense of womanhood. In some instances, the scars become permanent reminders of feelings of failure.

Arlene, Joan and Katie, all white middle- and upper middle-class women, represent a cluster within this study that has been able to retain the most lasting changes after their coronary event. Body image concerns and pressures to return to caretaking activities did not compromise these women's lives, as each resides somewhat outside the culturally prescribed gender identity for females. Arlene, who is divorced, lives with her mother in Maui and together they run a business. Her mother also experienced a heart attack, so they attended rehab together and now partake in exercise classes and cardiac support group meetings. Joan, who is married and has two grown children, runs a landscaping business, a typically male profession. She loves being physical on the job and working outdoors. Using Eastern philosophy and medicine, she and her strong group of female friends continue to educate themselves on health and wellness. Katie is a physical education teacher who lives with her lesbian partner, an academic. They both have radically altered their food to an extreme low-fat, high-fibre diet, and work out at the gym daily. They are also involved in women's health advocacy at a national level. By building lives outside the scope of more traditional female family arrangements, which also carry heavy cultural encumbrances such as the emphasis on women as caretakers, these females were able to formulate healthier choices and lifestyles.

## Discussion

### Relational processes and outcomes

For the analysis presented, the concept of 'gendered health synergies' (Sabo, 1999) helped us understand some of the relational processes and outcomes of the women and men we interviewed. Stated simply, the health of each sex is influenced by sociocultural synergies between the sexes. A *positive gendered health synergy* exists where the pattern of gender relations promotes favourable health processes or outcomes for both sexes. A *negative gendered health synergy* occurs where the pattern of gender relations is associated with unfavourable health processes or outcomes for one or both sexes. Consistent with critical feminist theories, the relations between men and women are also seen as unfolding within institutional contexts such as marriage, family, work, church and community. These 'gender regimes' (Connell, 1987) are further situated within the wider panoply of power relations and cultural meanings that reflect and reproduce interrelated gender, class and racial/ethnic inequalities.

To one extent or another, men's beliefs in the invulnerability of the male body fortified their denial of risk for CHD before diagnosis. Men played out the 'strong man' image in relation to women and children and in their own gender identities. The women in their lives, however, largely see through these men's masculine performances, and many interpreted men's 'sudden' heart attacks as a crashing down of men's pretensions. Ironically, these women's denial of their own susceptibility to develop CHD was masked by the biologistic assumption that heart disease is a 'men's disease'. Many of the women interviewed here construct a negative gendered health synergy, mobilised by wider patriarchal cultural myths that locate physical superiority and invulnerability within men's bodies and psychologies. The denial of both the women and men was embedded within these sexist beliefs.

Several gendered health synergies surrounded men's short-range and long-term recuperation from a coronary event and led generally to favourable outcomes. These outcomes were continuously mediated by complex interplays between social class, race and ethnicity. The men made attempts to reformulate their gender identities and change their lifestyles although, over time, many were not able to stick with all the changes. After the initial diagnosis shattered these men's masculine façades of invulnerability to illness and death, most of them became highly dependent on the women in their lives – spouses, children and relatives. With their independence compromised by disease, they more consciously surrendered to being cared for emotionally, physically and, in a few cases, economically. To varying degrees, they questioned those facets of their masculine identities that had emotionally distanced them from wives and family. They retreated from masculine assumptions about the invulnerability of the male body and cultural equations between masculine adequacy and emotional independence. In short, most of them got more in touch with their bodies and emotions, and reached out more to the women in their lives. In 'reaching out' to the women in their lives, for some men at least, there was a concomitant rethinking of masculinity that took the form of accepting physical vulnerability, 'slowing down', valuing what 'really matters in life', being less identified with work, and cherishing family and relationships. In effect, the men explored and embraced what are generally characterised within the gender binary of patriarchal culture as 'feminine' attributes or orientations. For the men, receiving care itself entailed some degree of accommodation to *being dependent* on others, and the 'others' were mainly women caregivers. Again, this involved making meaning outside prescribed gender relations.

Most of the women, in contrast, consciously avoided dependency on the men in their lives during the diagnosis and treatment phase. They were all concerned about the 'worry' they were 'causing' their husbands and children. These women put on a brave front while in the presence of their families, and sought out other sources of support that included other women such as sisters, close friends, co-workers and church group members. Whereas many of the men's psychosocial tendencies during the stormy period between diagnosis and treatment were to reach out to others for care and support, most of the women generally reached inward in order to mobilise the caretaker identity that was a large part of their pre-coronary lives as mothers, wives and women. Much of these women's immersion and psychosocial commitment to caretaking seemed consistent with more traditional cultural definitions of femininity and patterns of gender relations that revolve around being a nurturer. Indeed, part of these women's early denial that they would not fall victim to CHD was partly mobilised through the construction of the caretaker identity (i.e. 'I can't be the one to get sick because others need me' becomes 'I won't be the one to get sick because others need me'). Men's pre-coronary denial, in contrast, was fortified by quasi-conscious notions about physical toughness and the assumption that continuing to work or be physically active somehow meant immunity from heart disease.

## Relational dynamics and recovery

Treatment and recovery after the coronary event can be understood within a wider pattern of relational dynamics that are linked to caretaking and care-getting. Much of these women's discomfort with care-getting within the family appears to be partly mobilised by the centrality of their gender identity construction and investment in the emotional labour of care-giving. The construction of a caregiving identity and the channelling of women's emotional labour has often unfolded within marriage, family, kinship networks, and community. Within the sexual division of labour in many traditional families, the provision of emotional labour was mainly a feminine activity or orientation. Men's contribution to marital and family life was, traditionally, economic providership and provision of authority which, in turn, was often associated with emotional distance from wives and children. When men fell ill, they typically depended on the family for primary care and emotional sustenance which, again historically, was provided by women (Weis, 2004).

Most of the men interviewed in the current study experienced a disjuncture between the ways they constructed gender identity before, compared to after, their coronary event. The majority of them sought, and to varying degrees achieved, a post-coronary sense of direction in terms of emotional stability, by resuming activity through work or incorporating exercise and healthier eating habits into their lives. Many also reached out toward their loved ones as part of this reconstruction of their gender identity. While the males questioned aspects of their previous assumptions about masculinity and relationships, over time, all but a few reverted to some or all of their old ways. Two subgroups of women emerged within the sample we call 'traditionals' and 'non-traditionals'. The former refer to women who had prioritised marriage and family throughout their formative years, and they were heavily invested in the caretaker identity. The non-traditional women (about one-third of the sample) had careers and professional roles that, in many ways, operated outside the web of traditional relations. They enjoyed a network of women friends and associates, and men (even husbands) were not the primary source of nurturance and authentification in their lives.

During the phase of extended recovery for the non-traditional women, there was often continuity in regard to sticking with the identity construction of the caretaker from before the coronary event. The psychosocial assumption built into the reconstruction of the caretaking identity is that, by demonstrating to oneself and others that you are capable of caretaking, you are 'healthy' and 'back to normal'. For many women, the continuance of the caretaker identity was also fuelled by particular notions of guilt. During long-term recovery, these women expressed heavy layers of guilt emerging among the patterns of gender relations. During the initial treatment phase, many felt bad for putting their husbands and children through the ordeal and worry involved with their coronary event. These women said they felt guilty because they could have died and left their families motherless. Now with treatment behind them, many expressed guilt for not being able to successfully stick with all the needed lifestyle changes concerning diet and exercise. They cited lack of time to exercise and cook nutritious foods, while others lamented their return to stressful jobs outside the home. Many were keenly aware of sliding back into their dangerous habits. For these women, immersion in the caregiver and housewife-mother identities within their marriages and families complicated their personal recovery and attempts to redefine gender identity. Not only did the traditional females exhibit deep dimensions of guilt, but it was seemingly entwined with self-anger.

CHD created a fissure in these traditional women's life histories, and they tended to realign their gender identity construction with pre-coronary values and priorities, with the inclusion of a complex layer of guilt and anger. Men, in contrast, attempted with varying levels of success to question traditional masculine assumptions about the body and relationships in an effort to adopt a healthier lifestyle.

Whereas several of the women's long-term reconstruction of their body image revolved around issues pertaining to feminine beauty and body size, the men's efforts to redefine their post-coronary body emphasised returning to pre-coronary physical activities such as going back to work, being able to exercise and function sexually. Men's efforts to construct masculinity by 'doing' and, concomitantly, women's struggles to affirm themselves by 'appearing' attractive, reflect and reproduce wider patterns of gender relations within the western gender order. The gender theoretical aphorism seems to have explanatory relevance for our study; specifically, women are judged by how they look, men are judged by what they do.

An interesting theme emerged among the cluster of men and women who were positively able to transform their lives, bodies, and identities in profound and lasting ways. These men and women were solidly upper middle class, and therefore had relatively more resources, more education, access to better healthcare, and knowledge about how to get answers to health questions. The most successful men in our study were those who morphed their lives toward routine exercise, a better diet, less work stress, and closer relationships. Having held high-powered jobs, including owning large businesses, these men spent their lives immersed in busy days with long hours, and were former athletes and also involved in adventure sports and travel. After their coronary event, two of the three were able to retire altogether and 'focus on what was most important, family'. These preventive behaviours and lifestyle changes were partly facilitated by the rethinking of traditional masculinity. While two men in this subset were African American and one was white, the social and cultural resources available to those in the upper middle class was a powerful indicator in the ability for these males to reshape their lives and identity.

The subgroup of non-traditional women fared well through their post-coronary journey. They were white, upper middle class and, as previously described, lived their lives outside typical family models. Each was well educated, had good health coverage, and was savvy about the healthcare system. None of these women 'depended' on their husbands and family as much as others in our study for authentification through caretaking. It may be the case that many of the other women in the sample relied on maintaining the caretaker identity after their coronary event because they did not have the social and cultural resources to reconstruct their lives and identity as much as the more privileged women and men. Limited educational and social options may have resulted in a narrower and more concentrated investment in traditional femininity. They may simply not have had as many alternatives to work with in relation to the reconstruction of their new post-coronary identity. More hemmed in by traditional femininities, they had less social, personal and cultural 'clay on the wheel' to reconstruct gender identity and relations.

## Interactions of class, race and ethnicity

Finally, gender identity reconstructions after a coronary event were closely linked to interactions among social class, race and ethnicity. Among the men, the most favourable preventive health outcomes were experienced by the educated and more affluent subgroup, regardless of race and ethnicity, who seemed better able to reshape their lives and gender identity in healthy ways. Similarly, it was the non-traditional and upper middle-class women who had already developed more diversified modes of doing femininity who made healthful post-coronary adjustments. In contrast, healthful post-coronary re-adaptation was least likely to be an issue when racial and ethnic marginalisation merged with meagre socioeconomic resources. Most of the working-class and poor men, whether Native American, Hispanic or African American, did not have the social or subjective resources to orchestrate gender and lifestyle transformation during extended recovery (Sabo et al., 2006). Similarly, the long-term psychosocial adjustments of many of the traditional women in the sample were thwarted by economic deficits and a lack of alternative cultural options for expressing femininities.

While it may be an artefact of this sample, when comparing both the male and female participants, overall the female participants made less money, had less education, fewer savings and resources, and were more likely to be single due to divorce or death of a spouse. The women who were able to sidestep the negative facets of the caretaker identity exhibited two assets. Not only were they situated in upper middle-class social and cultural networks, but they also operated outside the cultural boundaries of traditional forms of female meaning-making altogether.

## Conclusion

Zierler and Krieger (1997) combined feminist theory with an analysis of political economy to explain the social production of disease among women. Our findings similarly suggest that the political economy of class, race and gender relations influences men's and women's long-term recovery from a coronary event. Class inequalities and cultural beliefs created positive and negative gender health synergies between men and women which, in turn, influenced their willingness and capacity to enact lifestyle changes, to manoeuvre through the health system, and to enjoy favourable psychosocial outcomes. More research on larger and diverse populations is needed to assess the accuracy and generalisability of our inferences.

## References

Addis, M.E. & Mahalik, J.R. (2003) Men, masculinity, and the contexts of help seeking. *American Psychologist*, **58**, 5–14.

Anyon, J. (2005) *Radical Possibilities: Public Policy, Urban Education, and a New Social Movement*. New York: Routledge.

Benz-Scott, L., Ben-Or, K. & Allen, J. (2002) Why are women missing from outpatient cardiac rehabilitation: should gender be considered? *Behavioral Medicine*, **27**, 149–166.

Bogdan, R. & Biklen, S. (2006) *Qualitative Research for Education: An Introduction to Theory and Methods.* 5th edn. Boston, MA: Allyn & Bacon.

Connell, R.W. (1987) *Gender and Power.* Stanford, CA: Stanford University Press.

Courtenay, W. (2000) Constructions of masculinity and their influence on men's well-being. *Social Science and Medicine,* **50**(10), 1385–1401.

Courtenay, W.H. (2002) A global perspective on the field of men's health: an editorial. *International Journal of Men's Health,* **1**(1), 1–13.

Edwards, M., Albert, N., Wang, C. & Apperson-Hansen, C. (2005) 1993–2003 gender differences in coronary artery revascularization: Has anything changed? *Journal of Cardiovascular Nursing,* **20**, 461–467.

Evans, R.E., Brotherstone, H., Miles, A. & Wardle, J. (2005) Gender differences in early detection of cancer. *Journal of Men's Health and Gender,* **2**(2), 209–217.

Farley, R., Wade, T. & Birchmore, L. (2003) Factors influencing attendance at cardiac rehabilitation among coronary heart disease patients. *European Journal of Cardiovascular Nursing,* **2**, 205–212.

Glaser, B. (1978) *Theoretical Sensitivity: Advances in the Methodology of Grounded Theory.* New York: Sociology Press.

Glaser, B. & Strauss, A. (1967) *Discovery of Grounded Theory: Strategies for Qualitative Research.* New York: Sociology Press.

Halm, M., Penque, S., Doll, W. & Beahrs, M. (1999) Women and cardiac rehabilitation patterns. *Journal of Cardiovascular Nursing,* **13**(3), 83–92.

Harrison, J., Chin, J. & Ficarrotto, T. (1992) Warning: masculinity may be dangerous to your health. In: *Men's Lives,* 2nd edn (eds M.S. Kimmel & M.A. Messner), pp.271–285. New York: Macmillan.

Jackson, L., Leclerc, J., Erskine, Y. & Linden, W. (2005) Getting the most out of cardiac rehabilitation: a review of referral and adherence predictors. *Heart,* **91**, 10–14.

Legato, M. (2000) Gender and the heart: sex-specific differences in normal anatomy and physiology. *Journal of Gender Specific Medicine,* **3**(7), 12–21.

McSweeny, J. & Coon, S. (2004) Women's inhibitors and facilitators associated with making behavioral changes after myocardial infraction. *MedSurg Nursing,* **13**, 49–56.

Payne, S. (2006) *The Health of Men and Women.* Cambridge: Polity Press.

Peddicord, K. (2005) Healthy hearts for women. *AWHONN Lifelines,* **9**, 35–38.

Sabo, D. (1999) *Understanding men's health: a relational and gender sensitive approach.* Harvard Center for Population and Development Studies. Working Paper Series Number 99.14. Available online: http://www.hsph.harvard.edu/Organizations/healthnet/HUpapers/gender/sabo.html

Sabo, D. (2005) The body politics of sports injury: culture, power, and the pain principle. In: *Sporting Bodies, Damaged Selves: Sociological Studies of Sports-Related Injury,* Vol. 2 (ed. K. Young), pp.59–80. London: Routledge.

Sabo, D., Hall, J. & Fix, G. (2006) Gender, denial, and men's lives after a coronary event. *Challenge: A Journal of Research on African American Men,* **12**(2).

Schofield, T., Connell, R.W., Walker, L., Wood, J. & Butland, D. (2000) Understanding men's health and illness: a gender relations approach to policy, research and practice. *Journal of American College Health,* **48**, 247–256.

Stanton, A. & Courtenay, W. (2003) Gender, stress and health. In: *Psychology Builds a Health World: Research and Practice Opportunities* (eds R.H. Rozensky, N.G.

Johnson, C.D. Goodheart & R. Hammond), pp.105–135. Washington, DC: American Psychological Association.

Thom, T., Haase, N., Rosamond, W. et al. (2006) Heart disease and stroke statistics—2006 update: a report from the American Heart Association Statistics Committee and Stroke Statistics Subcommittee. *Circulation*, **113**, 85–151.

Watson, J. (2000) *Male Bodies: Health, Culture and Identity*. Buckingham, UK: Open University Press.

Weis, L. (2004) *Class Reunion: The Remaking of the American White Working Class*. New York: Routledge.

Zierler, S. & Krieger, N. (1997) Reframing women's risk: social inequalities and HIV infection. *Annual Review of Public Health*, **18**(1), 401–436.

# Chapter 5

# SPECTACULAR RISK, PUBLIC HEALTH AND THE TECHNOLOGICAL MEDIATION OF THE SEXUAL PRACTICES OF GAY MEN

Mark Davis

## Introduction

This chapter critiques the framing of HIV risk-taking behaviour among gay men, with reference to popularised conceptions of risk-takers, research practice, and implications for public health. On a global scale, HIV overwhelmingly affects heterosexual people. In contrast, gay men are among the groups most affected in affluent countries, such as those in Europe, North America and Oceania, although this situation is changing. Because HIV prevalence is high, gay men have to make changes to their sexual and drug-using practices to avoid HIV infection. For those gay men who have HIV infection, there are additional concerns, such as: taking HIV treatment on a lifelong basis; informing partners, families and employers of their HIV serostatus, among other psychosocial concerns. Since the advent of the HIV epidemic in the early 1980s, gay men have made remarkable reductions in risk behaviour, partly through the action of individuals themselves, but also through community-based organisations in partnership with public health agencies. These changes in the sexual cultures of gay men are often heralded as good examples of how men's health could operate, at least in the domain of sexual health. However, research from the UK (Dodds et al., 2004), Australia (Prestage et al., 2005) and North America (Wolitski et al., 2001) has indicated that from 1996/7 reported risky sexual practice began to increase, suggesting that the practice of safer sex among gay men may have weakened. As I will discuss, attempts have been made to explain these changes, for example, the advent of antiviral treatment which is thought to reduce the perceived danger of HIV infection, and changes in the sexual cultures of gay men such as Internet-mediated partnering. None of these explanations on their own are convincing, with researchers resorting to the idea that changes in risk behaviour must be determined by some combination of all these factors. This position is itself somewhat unsatisfactory because it is unlikely that an effective explanation can be gained by combining insufficient ones.

However, one explanation of risk-taking has become central. This is the notion of 'barebacking' or the idea that some gay men might choose to have anal sex without condoms. From around the time that reported risk behaviour began to escalate, media commentators and HIV researchers began to document a practice where gay men appeared to engage in risky sexual intercourse knowing that it might transmit HIV, or even because it might do so. This idea of barebacking is used to draw attention to the transgression of safer sex guidelines. Barebacking also mobilises stereotypes of naturalised, unfettered male sexuality and the related repudiation of both self-care and regard for others in relation to HIV risk behaviour (Mane & Aggleton, 2001). It is no accident that such barebacking discourse arises in the face of increases in reported risk behaviour for which a satisfactory explanation is lacking. Because the idea of barebacking is regarded as transparently reprehensible and is partly anchored in stereotypes of male sexuality, it requires no explanation. It is an understanding of risk behaviour that is stripped of relational context and questions over the fallibility of both the method of safer sex and the conduct of the individual. It is thus rendered as a pure, volitional partaking of risk imbued with an understanding of sexual masculinity impervious to constraint. Such 'spectacular' risk is therefore the source of its own proof because it is risk-taking for risk-taking's sake. So purified, decontextualised and unfettered, this form of risk provides a touchstone in debate and research concerning risk practice and provides an alibi for public health struggling to connect with the sexual cultures of gay men.

The account of risk-taking discourse proposed here is not meant to deny that some gay men may choose, in certain situations and from time to time, to have sex that may transmit HIV. To do so would be to contradict over 20 years of research concerning responses to the risk of HIV transmission and living with HIV, some of which I will consider in the discussion to follow. Nor should this chapter be read as rejecting the idea that it is important to explore why reported risk practice has increased in recent years. This is an urgent issue for public health that also appears to be a problem in the area of injecting drug use (Hope et al., 2005). But this chapter does argue for a critically engaged public health that is reflexive about the cultural production of risk, risk-takers and risk practices. This perspective is not new. Some have argued that risk-taking of any kind needs to be addressed in cultural context (Lupton & Tulloch, 2002) and adopted this viewpoint to address the HIV epidemic (Lupton & Tulloch, 1998). I will draw on perspectives such as these in the discussion to follow. First, I explore the configuration of HIV risk-taking in popular media. Risk behaviour research will also be addressed, with reference to the illusory quality of a satisfactory social science explanation. I will then outline how the technologisation of the sexual cultures of gay men has become connected with the practice of barebacking. In the last section, I consider debates concerning barebacking in relation to the rise of individualism in tension with social obligation.

## Spectacular risk and public health

The idea that some gay men take risks on purpose has been the subject of some media excitement, particularly in the late 1990s. It seemed that the combination of sex, danger and errant citizenship was a story too good to refuse. I want to consider several interrelated dimensions of this spectacle of risk-taking: the narrative strategies that connect HIV risk-taking with the 'reality' genre of popular media; that such stories would not have been possible in earlier periods of the epidemic; and how such stories have revitalised panic discourse.

Commencing in 1997, there has been a flurry of barebacking stories, for example: in the gay men's print and online news media in the UK (Hoskins, 1999), Australia (Honnor, 1999) and the US (Scarce, 1999); the broadsheet media in the UK (Wells, 2000) and the US (Beswick, 2000); and online magazines (Freeman, 2003; Kennedy, 2006). The idea of transgressive risk-taking is a dominant theme in these stories, although not all of them have accepted barebacking discourse on face value. One article most ably mapped out the discursive organisation of barebacking as transgression (Signorile, 1997). The article depicted an Internet-relay-chat with a man seeking anal sex without condoms. Further, the chatter was said not to have known his HIV antibody serostatus, but was unconcerned because he believed that HIV treatments reduced the negative health consequences of HIV infection. This assemblage of mistaken knowledge and ethical failure has been characterised in various ways, for example: 'wilful' (Sheon & Plant, 2000); 'unapologetic' (Scarce, 1999). Other constructs include 'bug-chasing' and 'gift-giving', terms applied to men who seek HIV infection or who 'give' it (Laza, 2003). Importantly, some media stories have slid between unsafe sex between gay men with HIV to gay men with HIV spreading the HIV virus (Wells, 2000).

Barebacking stories make risk-taking visible, but they also represent a wider contestation of HIV prevention. The 1997 article exhibited doubtful ethics and epistemology in the practice of reporting on a single online chat as the basis for assertions concerning the reported behaviours of the chatter and others like him. It seems, however, that the apparent disregard for safer sex overshadowed any considerations of ethics or truth claims. Such stories represent a kind of 'post-political correctness' for the HIV epidemic coupled with 'tell it like it is' gusto. This approach resonates with the 'reality' genre of broadcast television. As Biressi and Nunn have pointed out, reality media, particularly that oriented to real crime stories, fuses drama and documentary, providing a tantalising, and sometimes nauseating, whirl of images and texts drawn from dramatised reconstructions, CCTV, mobile phone images, testimonials and moralising voice-overs (Biressi & Nunn, 2005). Like reality TV, barebacking stories draw together commentary, documentary and testimonial. The use of the Internet in sexual practice lends itself to this real crime approach because the products of cyber-culture, such as online chat, are easily collected. Assembled to focus on risk-taking, they provide ersatz reality TV feeds, or windows on what is 'really' happening out there. In addition, the adoption of the reality genre fits well with a generalised social conservatism concerning the moral degeneracy of late modern societies, often attributed to new technologies such as the Internet (Tomlinson, 1999). There is also reason to consider the voyeuristic qualities of barebacking stories (Denzin, 1995). As with TV programmes that rely on the reality genre (Biressi & Nunn, 2005), barebacking stories may provide a form of libidinal satisfaction for the audience. Readers can indulge in erotic, dangerous practice, without actually doing it. They can subscribe to a notion of themselves as ethically superior and pretend that barebacking is somehow restricted to the ethically defective, while at the same time partaking in the symbolic exchange of images of sexual hedonism and the rejection of risk reduction advice.

Barebacking stories are also historically specific. In early periods of the epidemic, the realisation that AIDS was caused by a sexually transmissible virus led to what was then called the AIDS crisis (Epstein, 1996). The crisis is said to have mobilised community action to alert gay men and drug users of the new danger and to encourage safer sex and sterile injecting drug use. One of the main reasons for community-based action was the reluctance of government to act. Public health was unable or unwilling to engage with stigmatised sexual and drug-using practices (Watney, 2000). In this early era of the AIDS crisis, it was not easy to raise moral outrage over unsafe sex, although of course, such a line of argument did appear in the mainstream press (see analysis of the British press on AIDS: Beharrell, 1993). But a moral outrage over unsafe sex was not easy to articulate because gay communities were consumed with responding to the threat of AIDS and caring for those who became ill, eking out meagre resources, and galvanising risk reduction practices among gay men and other affected groups. The rationality of HIV prevention concerned the encouragement of condom use where it had not been the norm. Barebacking stories reverse this rationality to draw attention to transgression of a normative condom use. It is possible, however, to recognise that the current outrage over barebacking was prefigured in this early period of community mobilisation. The invention of safer sex as a method and ethical stance on risk reduction was predicated on the stigma of some sexual and drug-using practices, the social status of affected communities, and the tardy action of government. It was inevitable then that, as these conditions softened and reformed in new ways, assumptions regarding the ethics of safer sex would also alter. Sontag presaged this situation in her discussion of the interplay of power and the biomedical management of the epidemic (Sontag, 1988). Sontag gestured towards a trajectory in the cultural engagement with HIV concerning the gradual focusing of requirements on conduct. In this light, barebacking panic stories represent a re-focusing of the practical and ethical management of the epidemic in relation to changes in the science and government that underpins it. Similarly, Treichler noted how a book called *AIDS: The Making of a Chronic Disease* was published in 1992, anticipating a hitherto unrealised end of the AIDS crisis (Treichler, 1999, p.325). Barebacking stories were waiting to be articulated and in all sorts of ways, social, biomedical and governmental changes have always had a relationship with the discursive management of HIV risk and sexual practice. The current valorisation of outrage regarding barebacking needs to be recognised as a specific, politicised configuration of HIV risk and sexual practice.

Barebacking stories also revitalise panic. In public health terms and at least in the affluent global North, HIV infection is now regarded as a chronic, manageable illness (Green & Smith, 2004). The introduction of effective HIV treatments in the mid 1990s and other improvements in the clinical management of HIV infection have resulted in this reappraisal of the symbolic and clinical status of HIV and AIDS. Further, media analyses of HIV and AIDS stories have identified the passing of the organising discourse of AIDS as crisis (Lupton, 1998). In light of these perspectives, barebacking stories can be seen as a turning back to panic discourse, resonant with the subsiding of AIDS as 'crisis' but modified for current circumstances. In this regard, such stories reveal a 'neo-crisis' rationality applied to risk, sex and identity. But in place of urgency concerning AIDS and the mobilisation of collective action to warn, protect and care, neo-crisis discourse is bound up with cynicism regarding the effectiveness of HIV prevention interventions and outrage concerning those gay men who are seen to be transgressing accepted sexual conduct.

## Measuring and explaining risky behaviour

Whether we see them as reactionary or necessary, neo-crisis stories concerning risk-taking wrap together the current issues for HIV prevention. In particular, they draw together concerns regarding how gay men engage with HIV prevention in relation to treatment-related changes in the status of HIV and AIDS and the emergence of the technological mediation of sexual partnering. Researchers have responded to this situation in an attempt to understand these changes. In this section, I will argue that the practice of barebacking disappears under social scientific scrutiny, revealing that we do not know very much about how gay men are negotiating the risk of HIV transmission in current circumstances. Researchers have difficulty arriving at a core definition of barebacking that captures the variety of understandings in circulation in the sexual cultures of gay men. However, they have identified so-called harm reduction strategies, such as sero-sorting and strategic positioning and related complexities.

A feature of barebacking is that it is not easily defined in behavioural terms, a problem that has both epistemological and public health implications. Wolitski has pointed out this problem in a review of risk behaviour research (Wolitski, 2007). He argues that while there is research that does explain anal sex without condoms, there is a lack of an explanation for the recent, historic increase in risk behaviour, especially concerning the notion that some gay men appear to 'consciously' reject safer sex. Wolitski provides a map of six factors that appear to be contributing to 'barebacking': the advent of HIV treatment; complex decision-making regarding HIV antibody serostatus and medical technologies; the advent of Internet-based sexual networking; drug use in and around sexual intercourse; safer sex fatigue; and changes in the scope and content of HIV prevention programmes. The problem with these explanations is that they also apply to anal sex without condoms in general. Wolitski also draws attention to the difficulties of defining barebacking in survey research, noting that researchers do not always agree. A recent survey of gay men appears to underscore these definitional problems. Huebner et al. (2006) asked gay men to categorise various sexual scenarios with terms including 'barebacking'. The respondents were found to refer to any anal sex without condoms as barebacking, that is, regardless of the intentions of the actors. Research participants are not alone in making this slippage from barebacking to any risky sexual practice. In another study, ostensibly exploring barebacking among gay men, Suarez and Miller (2001) enumerated the various social and psychological contexts of anal sex without condoms. This research suggests that scrutiny of barebacking leads back to the general case of the conditions of anal sex without condoms. In another example, researchers have linked barebacking to the cultural significance of the exchange of semen (Holmes & Warner, 2005). This notion has been discussed in previous research in relation to anal sex in general (Flowers et al., 1997). Likewise, psychotherapists working with gay men have attributed barebacking to psychosocial factors that, arguably, have been linked with anal sex without condoms in general (Shernoff, 2006; Cole, 2007).

Despite not being able to properly explain barebacking defined narrowly, research is revealing the variety of methods employed by gay men to reduce HIV transmission in situations where condoms are not used. Like others, Halkitis et al. (2007) in New York have reported that definitions of the practice of barebacking vary. However, gay men in their research appeared to be attempting to reduce the risk of anal sex without condoms through a practice of sero-sorting. Sero-sorting pertains to having anal sex without condoms with someone of (or assumed to be) the same HIV antibody status. Bimbi and Parsons (2007) have reported that male sex workers also appear to have adopted harm reduction strategies. In their commercial sex work, they appear to use a method that has been called 'strategic positioning', which means adopting a position in sexual intercourse that is thought to reduce the risk of HIV transmission. For example, gay men who know they have HIV might assume the receptive position in anal sex, which is thought to somewhat reduce HIV transmission (for a full discussion of strategic positioning and other risk reduction strategies, see Van de Ven et al., 2004).

Based on observations regarding the employment of risk reduction methods such as sero-sorting and positioning, researchers have begun to engage with harm reduction, an approach to illicit drug use that was established in the 1980s.[1] Briefly, harm reduction is a public health philosophy that established the practice of sterile injecting as a method for preventing

---

[1] See International Harm Reduction Association: www.ihra.net.

the transmission of HIV. Harm reduction creates a hierarchy of interventions that incorporates abstinence, addiction treatment and, for those who are not able or prepared to give up their drug use, access to methadone, needle exchanges and safe injecting rooms. Without such a hierarchy, it is believed that HIV prevention would not be effective as it would rely solely on abstinence and addiction treatment programmes. Commentators on barebacking have borrowed this idea to discuss how sero-sorting and positioning could become part of the repertoire of risk reduction methods used by gay men, alongside condoms. They argue that for those men who will not use condoms, forms of sero-sorting and positioning may provide some form of reduction of the risk of HIV transmission.

## Technologically mediated sexual cultures

Observations regarding sero-sorting and positioning suggest the importance of medical technologies in the sexual practices of gay men. In a discussion of medical technologies and safer sex, Flowers (2001) has pointed out how the HIV antibody test influences risk management practice by drawing attention to HIV in the body and therefore 'somatic' difference. Similarly, Lather (1995) has argued that the assignment of the antibody statuses of HIV-negative and HIV-positive create medical differences that mobilise kinds of risk relationships. Kippax and Race (2003) have discussed the complex ways in which gay men refer to HIV medical technologies to help them organise their sexual practices. The attention to the technological mediation of sexual practice resonates with the success of HIV treatment in terms of its effects on the virus in the body. Such biotechnical success reinforces a technological determinism in HIV prevention and research. Technological determinism can be taken to be a view regarding the relationship between society and technology that overestimates the contribution of technologies. Indeed, both HIV treatment and the Internet have been regarded as explanations for the rise in risky sex, as noted above. Despite qualifying evidence and argument, however, these technologies have been placed at the centre of research concerning gay men and risk behaviour. Further, although it is not often recognised, such research reveals that through the imperative of HIV prevention, Internet-mediated partnering and HIV medical technologies have become somewhat interdependent.

There has been research exploring the relationship between anal sex without condoms and Internet-mediated partnering in the US (Bull & McFarlane, 2000; Rhodes et al., 2002) and northern Europe (Hospers et al., 2002; Weatherburn et al., 2003). Similarly the impact of knowledge concerning HIV treatment has sponsored research in the UK, North America and Australia (Elford & Hart, 2005; International-Collaboration-on-HIV-Optimism, 2003). In general, this work does not support the techno-determinist view concerning risk behaviour. Research concerning the impact of treatment suggests that, while it may figure in the risk calculus of gay men, it does not explain the recent escalation of reported risky behaviour in different parts of the world (International-Collaboration-on-HIV-Optimism, 2003). In the UK, researchers used a repeated cross-sectional method to investigate treatment expectations over time among gay men (Elford et al., 2002). They found that while unsafe sex was associated with treatment expectations, the relationship remained constant over time, suggesting other factors (and not just treatment expectations) were contributing to the *escalation* of risky sex in the post-crisis situation.

Research concerning Internet-mediated sexual partnering shows that gay men are not more likely to have unprotected anal intercourse with their Internet partners compared with partners met in other ways (Bolding et al., 2005). It also appears that gay men use their profiles and online messages to sero-sort sexual partners (Carballo-Dieguez & Bauermeister, 2004; Dawson et al., 2005; Davis et al., 2006). Far less research has been done to assess the contribution of the Internet to risk behaviour among hetero-sexual people. Research suggests non-significant trends towards increased risk among women who use the Internet to find sex partners (Padgett, 2007). Research is also showing that compared with gay men, heterosexual men place far less emphasis on sexual health in their online communication regarding sexual activity (Phua et al., 2002). More research is needed to address these concerns, but it seems likely that gender relations will be important for the Internet-mediated sexual interaction among hetero-sexual people. In particular, the repudiation of sexual healthcare among heterosexual men and the resultant feminisation of such labour may be an important cultural frame for Internet-mediated sexual health.

What is not often considered, however, is the interdependent relation-ship between Internet-mediated partnering and medical technologies, and in particular how this relationship is forced into existence by the impera-tive of HIV prevention. For example, the question of barebacking articu-lated in Internet-mediated communication cannot arise without a pervasive requirement concerning safer sex. In addition, it is not possible to secure partners of the same (or assumed) serostatus via the Internet without some recourse to HIV diagnostic technologies that give rise to serostatus. These relationships are implicit in the research concerning Internet-mediated barebacking or implied in some research concerning barebacking *per se*. Much of this research appears to subscribe to a techno-determinist view that, as noted, has been found to lack support. But such research is valu-able because it signals the mingling of technologies in the sexual cultures of gay men. In addition, much like the media stories of barebacking already discussed, some researchers have begun analysing the products of mediated partnering, such as blogs and online profiles. Some of this research has a distinctly forensic turn. In this regard, terminology such as 'solicitation' in connection with Internet-mediated partnering and the pursuit of psycho-social 'profiling' of risk-takers appear to be significant. It may be that the real-crime genre I discussed in connection with the spectacle of risk is salient in such research activity. Some argue that barebacking is produced by Internet-mediated partnering in a rather condemning way (Gauthier & Forsyth, 1999). Others argue that the dehumanising qualities of new communications technologies contribute to the desire for bareback sex (Holmes et al., 2006). Apparently, the loneliness of the cyber age compels people to find intimacy in sex without condoms. Although arguing that there is little evidence for a causal link between advertising for bare-back partners and actual risky sex (Tewksbury, 2003), researchers have analysed the online profiles of people who espouse barebacking in an effort to 'profile' such people (Tewksbury, 2006). Others suggest that the so-called 'online barebacking phenomena' arises because some websites, overtly or otherwise, promote the idea that safer sex is a personal choice (Grov, 2006, p.995). In addition, the online mediation of barebacking dis-course is itself an epidemic, because of the dangerous 'exchange' of such discourses (Grov, 2004). These research approaches reflect the underlying anxiety related to both transgressive sex and technological innovation. But the online profiles and messages and other products of sexual cyber-culture so analysed nevertheless raise the prospect of the technologisation of sexual cultures of gay men in ways that are unfolding and for which we need improved descriptions.

The interdependency of technological mediation and medical technolo-gies is not complete, however. For example, what people say and do online may not be completely coherent with what happens offline and such lines of causation are difficult to establish in research. In addition, it is also possible that people who identify themselves as HIV-negative but suspect they are HIV-positive (because not recently tested) may behave differently than people who say and know they are HIV-negative. Such subtleties are yet to be thoroughly researched.

## Public health after 'barebacking'?

Researchers have begun to acknowledge sero-sorting and positioning as methods of harm reduction where condom use does not occur and to develop knowledge regarding the technological mediation of sex and risk management practice. But it appears that an effective social science explanation of narrowly defined barebacking is lacking and may not be useful given how the term is used in the sexual cultures of gay men. This problem is not surprising given that in contrast with anal sex without condoms in general, barebacking is defined in terms of the volitional transgression of safer sex. Several attempts have been made to address barebacking as the transgressive other of safer sex. Some of this analysis serves my previous observation concerning the spectacularisation of risk-taking. But these studies do converge on the notion that, because it forms an opposition with safer sex, the present focus on barebacking has to do with 'incorporating' it into HIV prevention. It is not so much reprehensible action that is at stake, but the refashioning of the rationality of safer sex to encapsulate various forms of engagement with the risk of HIV transmission, including barebacking. In this regard, the concept of harm reduction is currently being deployed as the method for such assimilation.

The notion of barebacking as transgression has been explored by several analysts. For example, Crossley (2004) used gay men's popular fiction to explore the supposed transgressive character of barebacking. Crossley appeared to argue that because homosexuality is a transgression of heteronormativity and that such transgression is laid down in the psyches of gay men, it should be no surprise that they transgress against public health guidelines. This supposed unconscious resistance of heteronormativity through a resistance of public health may be faulty because it elides heteronormativity and the good governance of sexual health, essentialises gay identity and leaves no room for an explanation of transgression on the part of heterosexual people (Flowers & Langdridge, 2007). Turning this notion of transgression in another, more interesting way, Riggs (2006) has argued that barebacking discourse is not properly understood as transgressive. This is because barebacking discourse reinforces the sanctioned status of adherence to public health guidelines and therefore actually reinforces heteronormativity. Riggs argued that, in contradistinction with Crossley, the outrage over barebacking provides a method for transferring the heterosex=good and homosex=bad duality to safer sex and barebacking, respectively. Riggs also argues that this duality of good sex/bad sex compels practices such as sero-sorting. Under 'heteronormative' governance of good sexual health, gay men are encouraged to find forms of sexual interaction that are not open to judgements of 'bad sex'. He therefore cautions against safer sex figured around HIV serostatus because such methods reinforce the administration of gay men's sexuality under heteronormative public health governance. But equally, given my previous comments with reference to HIV antibody testing, it is unlikely that there now exists a form of safer sex in which HIV serostatus does not figure. Also addressing the practice of barebacking, but in connection with reflections on other changes in the sexual cultures of gay men including the advent of HIV treatment and related technologies, Race (2003) has argued for a different view of barebacking. He makes the point that barebacking may be a form of code for HIV-positive serostatus and therefore a form of sero-sorting. In this view, barebacking coheres with a form of safer sex that is imbricated with the logic of the risk relationship produced by HIV antibody serostatus, as mentioned earlier. Barebacking is therefore derived from the combination of HIV medical technologies and the imperative of HIV prevention in the sexual cultures of gay men. In this regard, the practice of barebacking is patently not spectacular, nor is it decontextualised or even reprehensible. But Race also admits that barebacking as risk reduction is fragile and open to errors that have to do with, what he refers to as, disparities in knowledge and 'sexual capital'.

Another theme in the more theory-oriented research regarding barebacking concerns individualism and the supposed falling away of social obligation. Researchers in the US have argued that HIV prevention among gay men now draws on individualism (Sheon & Crosby, 2004, p.2117). Similarly, a researcher in Australia has argued that the notion of 'safer sex community' is no longer relevant for generations of gay men who made their sexual debut in the 1990s and 2000s (Ridge, 2004). In Canada and with specific reference to gay men who labelled themselves as barebackers, researchers have argued that a radically individualised risk negotiation is used by these men which hinges on the notion of caveat emptor (buyer beware) (Adam, 2005). Such negotiations are said to rely on a neo-liberal approach to civil society, which undercuts forms of mutual obligation.

The resort to individualism as an explanation of risk-taking needs to be set into the wider context of changes regarding the practice of public health. For example, researchers have argued that the dominant forms of HIV prevention speak to an individualised subject and therefore may imply individualism in the negotiation of safer sex (Dodds, 2002). In contrast and somewhat confusingly, public health in general refers to a notional expert patient who is assumed to be a risk-averse, rational actor (Ward et al., 2006). It may not be surprising therefore to find that individual sexual actors expect their partners to act in rational, self-protective ways. In this view, and in relation to practices such as sero-sorting, forgoing condoms may be taken as rational action in some situations. Bioethics in the area of HIV and infectious diseases is found to address an individualised, biological subject and therefore neglect social relations altogether (Tausig et al., 2006). These perspectives alert us to a dynamic in current public health practice that shifts risk responsibility onto the free, singular agents of liberal democracy with some unexpected and distinctly antithetical consequences for public health. In addition, it would be a mistake to assume that late modern forms of public health do not also retain an appeal to altruism. Drawing on Mauss and Titmuss, Waldby et al. (2004) have demonstrated, in relation to blood donation and the risk of infectious diseases, that donors recognised the value of both prudent action in terms of the healthy self and giving to strangers. This research also demonstrates that public health is more properly considered as a flux of individualism and social obligation open to reconfiguration, partly in relation to changes in scientific knowledge and technological innovation. In this regard, the barebacking/safer sex duality is the spectacular form of such politics in the area of HIV, itself undergoing radical changes related to medical and other technologies. Less sensational but more significant are recent interventions, particularly for people with HIV, that have stressed responsible action on the part of individuals inside a general framing of their obligations to avoid HIV transmission and therefore the protection of the community in abstract. Recent policy has advocated altruism as a basis for HIV prevention among people with HIV. In some versions, HIV prevention altruism centres on the cultivation of responsibility for avoiding transmission of HIV to sexual partners (Janssen et al., 2001). A recent US multi-city campaign aimed to bolster responsible action on the part of individuals with HIV.[2] Somewhat revising altruism, the National Association of People with AIDS (NAPWA) in the US has formulated guidelines that recognise how altruism and autonomy can be combined in HIV prevention work, defining sexual health in terms of the capacity of people with HIV to be able to articulate their needs and act on them.[3] In the UK and Australia, HIV prevention frameworks have similarly emphasised the autonomy of people with HIV (Ward, 2001; Triffitt & People-Living-With-HIV/AIDS, 2004). Elsewhere, I have questioned the idea of a straightforward hyper-individualism and loss of community in HIV prevention (Davis, 2008). In this research, interviewees were focused on resisting the blame that could be attached to HIV-positive sero-identity. In this view, practices of sero-sorting emerged as one possible method for reducing such pressures in sexual practice.

---

[2] See www.hivstopswithme.org.
[3] See www.napwa.org.

## Conclusion

In this chapter, I have made connections between the spectacle of risk-taking, how it is defined and understood, and its involvement in the technologisation of the sexual cultures of gay men. I have argued that such connections enable a different viewpoint for the current turn in the debate and research concerning risk-taking behaviour among gay men.

I have suggested that the popular framing of risk-taking represents anxieties concerning changes in the sexual practices of gay men, tinged with voyeuristic satisfaction. Such stories are fashioned to reveal a purely volitional form of risk-taking that also relies on notions of the repudiation of self-care and regard for others that figure in stereotypical notions of male sexuality. This spectacularisation of a specific form of risk-taking appears to provide the means for identifying errant citizens, defined not in terms of their fallibility or lack of awareness, but in terms of their enjoyment of risk. This spectacle of risk also has the effect of constituting risk culture so that it deflects attention away from the fallibility of institutional practices such as those of public health.

In relation to barebacking, researchers have also begun to document an important separation in the concepts of barebacking in circulation in gay men's sexual cultures and reductive social science definitions. In contrast with the spectacle of risk and risk behaviour research, gay men themselves use the term barebacking in a variety of ways, including as a generic handle for any anal sex without condoms. Researchers themselves have revealed the difficulties of explaining barebacking, often with recourse to psycho-social conceptualisations of risk behaviour that apply to anal sex without condoms in general. Although it has shown that gay men may be using forms of 'harm reduction' such as sero-sorting and positioning, I have suggested that research driven by the spectacle of risk, and therefore focusing on narrowly defined volitional risk-taking, does not yield very much in terms of explanation. This splitting of both epistemology and public health from the life worlds of citizens has serious implications for HIV/AIDS and possibly for other health concerns.

In concert with risk behaviour research, analysts have tried to understand risk-taking in cultural terms, exploring barebacking as transgression of public health, as constitutive of heteronormativity, or both. By implication, this research has raised the so far unresolved concern to do with the extent to which HIV prevention can incorporate barebacking and the related methods of sero-sorting and positioning inside a rubric of harm reduction for sexual health. It has also begun to map out a tension in public health concerning the clashing of individualism with social obligation.

While other areas of healthcare become thoroughly engaged with a biologised, atomised, prudent subject, public health in the area of HIV and other sexually transmitted diseases necessarily relies on the obligations of subjects to act to some extent for the good of their sexual partners and, through them, for the good of the social. This rationality is most often expressed as a required altruism on the part of gay men with HIV. There are dangers in making people with HIV solely responsible for HIV prevention. But it may also be the case that without altruism and in the context of an increasingly individualised system of healthcare, public health governance will resort to containment and quarantine, traditions that have always ghosted responses to HIV. Indeed, for not practising safer sex, people with HIV have been convicted of grievous bodily harm in England and elsewhere in the UK (Dodds & Keogh, 2006) and in other countries (Nyambe et al., 2005). As I noted also, some research regarding barebacking has a somewhat forensic flavour, possibly an expression of this turning to containment in public health for HIV. This dynamic of individualism, altruism and coercion has serious implications for HIV and public health in general.

The other main theme of this chapter has been the technologisation of sexual practice, in particular: Internet-mediated sero-sorting, strategic positioning and other complexities. While I cautioned against a rush to techno over-determinacy, such research does underline the involvement of an assemblage of technologies and public health rationalities in the sexual cultures of gay men, particularly with regard to the ways that the imperative of HIV prevention forces relationships between Internet-mediated partnering and HIV serostatus, among others. To be useful for gay men in connection with HIV and for citizens in relation to health in general, public health requires some reflection on its own involvement in the constitution of risk, risk-takers and risk-taking.

## Acknowledgement

For their helpful comments on drafts of this chapter, I would like to thank Professor Corinne Squire of the University of East London and Professor Paul Flowers of Glasgow Caledonian University.

## References

Adam, B. (2005) Constructing the neoliberal sexual actor: responsibility and care of the self in the discourse of barebackers. *Culture, Health and Sexuality*, 7(4), 333–346.
Beharrell, P. (1993) AIDS and the British Press. In: *Getting the Message* (ed. J. Eldridge). London: Routledge.

Beswick, T. (2000) Bareback 'outings' spark debate over well-known secret. *Bay Area Reporter*, San Francisco.

Bimbi, D. & Parsons, J. (2007) Barebacking among Internet based male sex workers. In: *Barebacking: Psychosocial and Public Health Approaches* (eds P. Halkitis, L. Wilton & J. Drescher). New York: Haworth Medical Press.

Biressi, A. & Nunn, H. (2005) *Reality TV: Realism and Revelation.* London: Wallflower Press.

Bolding, G., Davis, M., Hart, G., Sherr, L. & Elford, J. (2005) Gay men who look for sex on the Internet: is there more HIV/STI risk with online partners? *AIDS*, **19**, 961–968.

Bull, S. & McFarlane, M. (2000) Soliciting sex on the Internet: what are the risks for sexually transmitted diseases and HIV? *Sexually Transmitted Diseases*, **27**(9), 545–550.

Carballo-Dieguez, A. & Bauermeister, J. (2004) 'Barebacking': intentional condomless anal sex in HIV-risk contexts: reasons for and against it. *Journal of Homosexuality*, **47**(1), 1–16.

Cole, G. (2007) Barebacking: transformations, dissociations and the theatre of counter-transference. *Studies in Gender and Sexuality*, **8**(1), 49–68.

Crossley, M. (2004) Making sense of 'barebacking': gay men's narratives, unsafe sex and the 'resistance habitus'. *British Journal of Social Psychology*, **43**, 225–244.

Davis, M. (2008) The 'loss of community' and other problems for sexual citizenship in recent HIV prevention. *Sociology of Health and Illness*, **30**(2), 182–196.

Davis, M., Hart, G., Bolding, G., Sherr, L. & Elford, J. (2006) E-dating, identity and HIV prevention: theorising sexual interaction, risk and network society. *Sociology of Health and Illness*, **28**(4), 457–478.

Dawson, A.G. Jr, Ross, M.W., Henry, D. & Freeman, A. (2005) Evidence of HIV transmission risk in barebacking men-who-have-sex-with-men: cases from the Internet. *Journal of Gay & Lesbian Psychotherapy*, **9**, 73–83.

Denzin, N. (1995) *The Cinematic Society: The Voyeur's Gaze.* London: Sage Publications.

Dodds, C. (2002) Messages of responsibility: HIV/AIDS prevention materials in England. *Health: An Interdisciplinary Journal for the Social Study of Health, Illness and Medicine*, **6**(2), 139–171.

Dodds, C. & Keogh, P. (2006) Criminal prosecutions for HIV transmission: people living with HIV respond. *International Journal of STD and AIDS*, **17**(5), 315–318.

Dodds, J., Mercey, D., Parry, J. & Johnson, A. (2004) Increasing risk behaviour and high levels of undiagnosed HIV infection in a community sample of homosexual men. *Sexually Transmitted Infections*, **80**, 236–240.

Elford, J. & Hart, G. (2005) HAART, viral load and sexual risk behaviour. *AIDS*, **19**, 205–207.

Elford, J., Bolding, G. & Sherr, L. (2002) High-risk sexual behaviour increase among London gay men between 1998 and 2001: what is the role of HIV optimism? *AIDS*, **16**, 1–8.

Epstein, S. (ed.) (1996) *Impure Science: AIDS, Activism and the Politics of Knowledge.* Berkeley, CA: University of California Press.

Flowers, P. (2001) Gay men and HIV/AIDS risk management. *Health*, **5**, 50–75.

Flowers, P. & Langdridge, D. (2007) Offending the other: deconstructing narratives of deviance and pathology. *British Journal of Social Psychology*, **46**(3), 679–690.

Flowers, P., Smith, J., Sheeran, P. & Beail, N. (1997) Health and romance: understanding unprotected sex in relationships between gay men. *British Journal of Health Psychology*, **2**, 73–86.

Freeman, G. (2003) In search of death: Bug chasers: the men who long to be HIV+. *Rolling Stone.* Digital edition: www.rollingstone.com. Published 23 January. Accessed 14 August 2007.

Gauthier, D. & Forsyth, C. (1999) Bareback sex, bug chasers and the gift of death. *Deviant Behaviour*, **20**, 85–100.

Green, G. & Smith, R. (2004) The psychosocial and health care needs of HIV-positive people in the United Kingdom following HAART: a review. *HIV Medicine*, **5**(Suppl 1), 1–46.

Grov, C. (2004) 'Make me your death slave': men who have sex with men and use the Internet to intentionally spread HIV. *Deviant Behaviour*, **25**(4), 329–349.

Grov, C. (2006) Barebacking websites: electronic environments for reducing or inducing HIV risk. *AIDS Care*, **18**(8), 990–997.

Halkitis, P., Wilton, L. & Galatowitsch, P. (2007) What's in a term? How gay and bisexual men understand barebacking. In: *Barebacking: Psychosocial and Public Health Approaches* (eds P. Halkitis, L. Wilton & J. Drescher). New York: Haworth Medical Press.

Holmes, D. & Warner, D. (2005) The anatomy of a forbidden desire: men, penetration and semen exchange. *Nursing Inquiry*, **12**(1), 10–20.

Holmes, D., O'Byrne, P. & Gastaldo, D. (2006) Raw sex as limit experience: a Foucauldian analysis of unsafe anal sex between men. *Social Theory & Health*, **4**(4), 319–333.

Honnor, G. (1999) Do you jackaroot? *Sydney Star Observer*, Sydney.

Hope, V., Judd, A., Hickman, M., Sutton, A., Stimson, G., Parry, J. & Gill, N. (2005) HIV prevalence among injecting drug users in England and Wales 1990 to 2003: evidence for increased transmission in recent years. *AIDS*, **19**(11), 1207–1214.

Hoskins, M. (1999) Bareback on the net. *Positive Nation*, 26–28.

Hospers, H., Harterink, P., van den Hoek, K. & Veenstra, J. (2002) Chatters on the Internet: a special target group for HIV prevention. *AIDS Care*, **14**(4), 539–544.

Huebner, D.M., Proescholdbell, R.J. & Nemeroff, C.J. (2006) Do gay and bisexual men share researchers' definitions of barebacking? *Journal of Psychology & Human Sexuality*, **18**(1), 67–77.

International-Collaboration-on-HIV-Optimism (2003) HIV treatments optimism among gay men: an international perspective. *Journal of Acquired Immune Deficiency Syndromes*, **32**, 545–550.

Janssen, R., Holtgrave, D., Valdiserri, R., Shepherd, M., Gayle, H. & De Cock, K. (2001) The serostatus approach to fighting the HIV epidemic: prevention strategies for infected individuals. *American Journal of Public Health*, **91**(7), 1019–1024.

Kennedy, S. (2006) 'They're peddling death'. *The Advocate*, Digital Edition, www.advocate.com. Accessed 14 August 2007.

Kippax, S. & Race, K. (2003) Sustaining safe practice: twenty years on. *Social Science and Medicine*, **57**, 1–12.

Lather, P. (1995) The validity of angels: interpretive and textual strategies in researching the lives of women with HIV/AIDS. *Qualitative Inquiry*, **1**(1), 41–68.

Laza, M. (2003) Bug chasing. *The Mail on Sunday*.

Lupton, D. (1998) The end of AIDS?: AIDS reporting in the Australian press in the mid-1990s. *Critical Public Health*, **8**(1), 33–46.

Lupton, D. & Tulloch, J. (1998) The adolescent 'unfinished body', reflexivity and HIV/AIDS risk. *Body and Society*, **4**(2), 19–34.

Lupton, D. & Tulloch, J. (2002) 'Life would be pretty dull without risk': voluntary risk-taking and its pleasures. *Health, Risk and Society*, **4**(2), 113–124.

Mane, P. & Aggleton, P. (2001) Gender and HIV/AIDS: What do men have to do with it? *Current Sociology*, **49**(6), 23–37.

Nyambe, M., Gaines, H. & Yocum, T. (2005) *Criminalisation of HIV transmission in Europe: draft*. Global Network of People Living with HIV/AIDS (Europe) and Terrence Higgins Trust.

Padgett, P. (2007) Personal safety and sexual safety for women using online personal ads. *Sexuality Research & Social Policy*, **4**(2), 27–37.

Phua, V., Hopper, J. & Vazquez, O. (2002) Men's concerns with sex and health in personal advertisements. *Culture, Health & Sexuality*, **4**(3), 355–363.

Prestage, G., Mao, L., Fogarty, A., Van de Ven, P., Kippax, S., Crawford, J., Rawstorne, P., Kaldor, J., Jin, F. & Grulich, A. (2005) How has the sexual behaviour of gay men changed since the onset of AIDS: 1986–2003. *Australian and New Zealand Journal of Public Health*, **29**(6), 530–535.

Race, K. (2003) Revaluation of risk among gay men. *AIDS Education and Prevention*, **15**(4), 369–381.

Rhodes, S., DiClemente, R., Cecil, H., Hergenrather, K. & Yee, L. (2002) Risk among men who have sex with men in the United States: a comparison of an Internet sample and a conventional outreach sample. *AIDS Education and Prevention*, **14**(1), 41–50.

Ridge, D. (2004) 'It was an incredible thrill': the social meanings and dynamics of younger gay men's experiences of barebacking in Melbourne. *Sexualities*, **7**(3), 259–279.

Riggs, D. (2006) 'Serosameness' or 'serodifference'? Resisting polarised discourse of identity and relationality in the context of HIV. *Sexualities*, **9**(4), 409–422.

Scarce, M. (1999) A ride on the wild side. *POZ Magazine*.

Sheon, N. & Crosby, M. (2004) Ambivalent tales of HIV disclosure in San Francisco. *Social Science and Medicine*, **58**, 2105–2118.

Sheon, N. & Plant, A. (2000) Protease dis-inhibitors? The gay bareback phenomenon. www.managingdesire.org/sexpanic/ProteaseDisinhibitors.html.

Shernoff, M. (2006) Condomless sex: gay men, barebacking and harm reduction. *Social Work*, **51**(2), 106–113.

Signorile, M. (1997) Bareback and restless. http://www.signorile.com/articles/outbbr.html

Sontag, S. (1988) *AIDS and its Metaphors*. London: Penguin.

Suarez, T. & Miller, J. (2001) Negotiating risks in context: a perspective on unprotected anal intercourse and barebacking among men who have sex with men – where do we go from here? *Archives of Sexual Behaviour*, **30**(3), 287–300.

Tausig, M., Selgelid, M., Subedi, S. & Subedi, J. (2006) Taking sociology seriously: a new approach to the bioethical problems of infectious disease. *Sociology of Health & Illness*, **28**(6), 838–849.

Tewksbury, R. (2003) Bareback sex and the quest for HIV: assessing the relationship in Internet personal advertisements of men who have sex with men. *Deviant Behaviour*, **24**(5), 467–482.

Tewksbury, R. (2006) 'Click here for HIV': an analysis of Internet-based bug chasers and bug givers. *Deviant Behaviour*, **27**(4), 379–395.

Tomlinson, J. (1999) *Globalisation and Culture*. Cambridge: Polity Press.

Treichler, P. (1999) *How to Have Theory in an Epidemic: Cultural Chronicles of AIDS*. Durham, NC: Duke University Press.

Triffitt, K. & People-Living-With-HIV/AIDS (2004) *Let's Talk About It: Me, You and Sex*. Sydney, Australia: People Living with HIV/AIDS, New South Wales.

Van de Ven, P., Murphy, D., Hull, P., Prestage, G., Batrouney, C. & Kippax, S. (2004) Risk management and harm reduction among gay men in Sydney. *Critical Public Health*, **14**(4), 361–376.

Waldby, C., Rosengarten, M., Treloar, C. & Fraser, S. (2004) Blood and bioidentity: ideas about self, boundaries and risk among blood donors and people living with hepatitis C. *Social Science and Medicine*, **59**(7), 1461–1471.

Ward, K., Davis, M. & Flowers, P. (2006) Patient expertise and innovative health technologies. In: *Innovative Health Technologies, Health Technology and Society Series* (ed. A. Webster). Basingstoke, UK: Palgrave Macmillan.

Ward, M. (2001) Making it better: guiding principles for the inclusion of the needs and rights of gay men with HIV in sexual health promotion and primary HIV prevention. London: Network of Self Help and HIV & AIDS Groups.

Watney, S. (2000) *Imagine Hope: AIDS and Gay Identity*. London: Routledge.

Weatherburn, P., Hickson, F. & Reid, D. (2003) *Net Benefits: Gay Men's Use of the Internet and Other Settings where HIV Prevention Occurs*. London: Sigma Research.

Wells, M. (2000) Sex on the edge. *The Guardian*, London.

Wolitski, R. (2007) The emergence of barebacking among gay and bisexual men in the United States: a public health perspective. In: *Barebacking: Psychosocial and Public Health Approaches* (eds P. Halkitis, L. Wilton & J. Drescher). New York: Haworth Medical Press.

Wolitski, R., Valdiserri, R., Denning, P. & Levine, W. (2001) Are we headed for a resurgence of the HIV epidemic among men who have sex with men? *American Journal of Public Health*, **91**(6), 883–888.

# Chapter 6

# YOUNG MEN, MASCULINITY AND ALCOHOL

Richard de Visser

## Introduction

There is widespread concern about the health and social consequences of excessive alcohol consumption among young men (Rehm et al., 2001; Prime Minister's Strategy Unit [PMSU], 2004; Department of Health [DoH], 2007). Binge drinking is by no means restricted to young men, but in developed western nations young adult men are more likely than other people to binge drink (Kuntsche et al., 2004; de Visser et al., 2006; DoH, 2007). The aim of this chapter is to give an overview of rates and correlates of binge drinking among young men. This chapter begins with a brief overview of the range of possible influences on young men's alcohol consumption and then moves to a focus on the interplay between cultural ideologies of masculinity and young men's drinking.

## Young men's alcohol consumption

Different definitions of binge drinking have been employed in different countries and in different research studies. Some define binge drinking as consumption of a certain quantity of alcohol in one day or drinking session (de Visser et al., 2006; Andersson et al., 2007; DoH, 2007); others have used more qualitative definitions such as 'fast and excessive drinking' (Hammersley & Ditton, 2005); while other studies have drawn from both definitions (see for example Ministry of Health, 2007).

Regardless of the definition used, it is clear that many young men binge drink and that young men are more likely than other population groups to binge drink. This pattern is found in Australia (de Visser et al., 2006; Andersson et al., 2007), Britain (Lader & Goddard, 2006), New Zealand (Ministry of Health, 2007), and the United States (Wechsler et al., 2002;

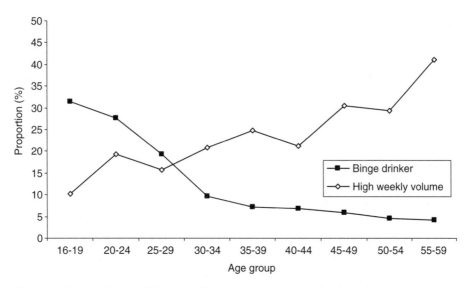

**Figure 6.1** Prevalence of binge drinking and excessive weekly alcohol consumption in a population-representative sample of Australian men.

Substance Abuse and Mental Health Services Administration, 2004), as well as in cross-national European research (Kuntsche et al., 2004). For example, data from the Australian Study of Health and Relationships (ASHR) (de Visser et al., 2006) showed that young men were more likely than other members of the population to binge drink and to engage in several other health risk behaviours. Figure 6.1 above shows clear age-related trends in both binge drinking (i.e. seven or more 10g units of alcohol in one session) and excessive weekly alcohol consumption (i.e. 29 or more 10g units of alcohol in one week) in the ASHR data. Data such as these suggest that, although younger men's overall volume of alcohol consumption tends to be lower than that of older men, this volume of consumption is concentrated in fewer drinking sessions. Indeed, nearly all of young men's alcohol consumption occurs in binge-drinking sessions, whereas older men tend to drink more frequently but consume less on each drinking day (Stockwell et al., 2002).

There are clear health and social consequences associated with binge drinking (Rehm et al., 2001; PMSU, 2004). People who binge drink are: at increased risk of alcohol poisoning; more likely to be involved in accidents (including road traffic accidents); more likely to sustain injuries; and more likely to be the victims or perpetrators of violence. Added to these individual health consequences is the interpersonal, social and financial costs of excessive alcohol consumption. Excessive alcohol consumption among young men is also a concern because it predicts binge drinking during adulthood (Jefferis et al., 2005). Concern about excessive alcohol consumption among young men demands an understanding of why some young men drink excessively, while other men drink moderately or not at all. Such information may facilitate the development of interventions to reduce excessive alcohol consumption and its associated health and social costs.

## Influences on young men's drinking

It is important to consider how demographic, social and attitudinal factors interact to influence men's alcohol consumption. For example, levels of binge drinking vary according to ethnicity. Data from the United States and United Kingdom reveal that excessive alcohol use is more common among white young adults than among other ethnic/racial groups, particularly compared with young black men (Best et al., 2001; Wechsler et al., 2002; Heim et al., 2004; Pugh & Bry, 2007). However, ethnic minority youth are more likely to drink if they have friends within their ethnic community who drink or friends outside their ethnic group (Heim et al., 2004) and if they have a weaker 'ethnic identity' (Pugh & Bry, 2007).

Socioeconomic factors may also influence binge drinking among young men. In the general population, binge drinking is associated with lower socioeconomic status (Droomers et al., 1999), and unemployment has been found to contribute to the development of problem drinking (Claussen, 1999). However, among young adults there is less consistent evidence for a link between socioeconomic status and binge drinking (Muthén & Muthén, 2000; McCarthy et al., 2002; Casswell et al., 2003; de Visser et al., 2006; Hanson & Chen, 2007). Measurement of socioeconomic status may be particularly difficult among young men because they are in a transitional phase in which socioeconomic status measures, such as education or personal income, may not accurately reflect family background or final adult destinations (de Visser et al., 2006).

Perceptions of peer drinking norms (Perkins, 2002; Johnston & White, 2003) and peer influences (Kuntsche et al., 2004) affect young people's alcohol consumption. Young people are more likely to binge drink if they think that more of their peers binge drink (and many mistakenly believe that more of their peers drink than actually do), or if they have experienced encouragement or pressure to binge drink. Recent research has also shown that adolescents' perceptions of peers who drink mediate the influence of peer and parental norms on adolescents' alcohol use (Spijkerman et al., 2007).

Drinking behaviour is also influenced by personality (Caspi et al., 1997; Kuntsche et al., 2004), attitudes (Wardle & Steptoe, 2003) and future-orientation (Henson et al., 2006). The high prevalence of binge drinking among young men is also influenced by sex differences in reasons for drinking and expectancies related to alcohol consumption (Rauch & Bryant, 2000; Borjesson & Dunn, 2001). For example, a stronger motive of 'drinking to get drunk' predicts binge drinking in young adults, and men are more likely than women to endorse this motive (Schulenberg et al., 1996). In addition, problematic alcohol use is more common among men with a lower sense of control over their lives (McCreary et al., 1999).

## The importance of masculinity

The studies referred to above indicate that, among young men, different psychosocial factors influence which men will binge drink and which will not. Gender and gender roles are another potentially important influence on young men's drinking which can be conceptualised at both an individual and a social level. The observation that young men are more likely than other people to drink excessively is sometimes interpreted as implying that masculinity or 'maleness' are inherently problematic. This is not surprising given the finding that men are more likely to engage in a range of health-compromising behaviours, and less likely to engage in health-protective or health-promoting behaviours (Courtenay, 2000). However, if there were simple links between masculinity, alcohol consumption and binge drinking, then we could not explain why many men drink moderately or abstain from alcohol.

Alcohol research frequently examines sex differences (male/female), but not gender differences (masculine/feminine). Such research cannot determine why, or how, masculinity influences some young men to drink excessively while others do not. However, there is a need for such information in order to understand the interplay between gender and health-related behaviours (Courtenay, 2000). Although masculinity has been identified as an important influence on health-related behaviour, little is known about how ideologies of masculinity are enacted by *individual* men via *particular* behaviours within *particular* social contexts (Courtenay, 2000).

Gender double standards towards drinking and drunkenness are important influences on sex differences in alcohol use (Lemle & Mishkind, 1989; Leigh, 1995). It has been suggested that heavy drinking is symbolic of masculinity because it is linked to other aspects of traditional masculine roles such as unconventionality, risk-taking and aggression, whereas heavy drinking among women is not condoned as it is linked to unwomanly behaviour such as sexual disinhibition, and perceived to impair nurturing, maternal behaviour (Lemle & Mishkind, 1989; Leigh, 1995; Plant et al., 2002; Mullen et al., 2007). Being able to drink excessively and to 'hold one's drink' are important elements of traditional masculinity (de Visser & Smith, 2007a; Plant et al., 2002), but there are very few social spaces in which excessive drinking by women is condoned (Montemurro & McClure, 2005).

The equation of drinking and masculinity is reflected in the observation that women who binge drink are presented in the media as unfeminine, as wanting to be like men, and as emasculating through their appropriation of masculine behaviour (Day et al., 2004; Jackson & Tinkler, 2007). Indeed, terms used to describe young women who binge drink – for example, 'ladette' and 'bachelorette' – are feminised versions of terms used to describe men (Day et al., 2004; Montemurro & McClure, 2005; Jackson & Tinkler, 2007). Any positive representations of women's public drinking relate it to the traditionally male domains of professionalism, public life, adventure and risk (Lyons et al., 2006). In addition to reinforcing differences in *how* men and women drink, media and marketing perpetuate gendered distinctions between appropriate men's and women's drinks (McCreanor et al., 2005; Lyons et al., 2006).

### Interaction of sex and gender roles

Whatever the magnitude of any observed sex differences in alcohol consumption, it is important to note that different patterns of alcohol use in men and women are not simply sex differences. Sex differences in drinking are mediated by gender role attributes and attitudes (Huselid & Cooper, 1992; McCreary et al., 1999; Ricciardelli et al., 2001; Williams & Ricciardelli, 2003; Nolen-Hoeksema, 2004; van Gundy et al., 2005). Among women *and* men, higher levels of alcohol consumption are related to negative 'masculine' characteristics such as aggression, and among both women *and* men, lower levels of alcohol consumption are related to positive 'masculine' characteristics such as instrumentality, and positive 'feminine' characteristics such as nurturance. Different configurations of gender role attitudes are related to different patterns of alcohol consumption, and there are not simple links between masculinity/femininity and alcohol consumption (McCreary et al., 1999; Mahalik et al., 2006; Mullen et al., 2007). It is important, therefore, to examine how young men experience the links between their sex, their gender identity and their alcohol consumption.

## Masculine identities and health-related behaviour

Although gender stereotypes of alcohol use and binge drinking exist, it is important to note that there are not simple links between masculinity and alcohol consumption. Rather than there being one single masculinity, there exist several different ways of being masculine (Connell, 1995; Edley & Wetherell, 1997; Frosh et al., 2002; Kimmel & Messner, 2003). Many men endorse and aspire to 'hegemonic masculinity' (Connell, 1987, 1995), the dominant discourse of masculinity characterised by physical and emotional toughness, risk-taking, predatory heterosexuality, being the breadwinner, and so on. Although different versions of masculinity exist, not all masculinities are equally valued: hegemonic masculinity (i.e. traditional or conventional masculinity) has greater legitimacy and power than alternative forms (for example, new-age men and 'metrosexuals'). Indeed, it has been noted that in constructing non-hegemonic masculinities, men must navigate between 'the Scylla of the macho man and the Charybdis of the wimp' (Edley & Wetherell, 1997, p.211).

Behavioural elements of hegemonic masculinity are commonly set up in binary opposition to their alternatives, so that anything other than the hegemonic form is immediately non-masculine (see for example McQueen & Henwood, 2002). Positioning theory (Harré & van Langenhove, 1998) proposes that individuals actively create identities by positioning themselves (or being positioned) in relation to dominant and subordinate discourses in their cultural context. This positioning facilitates or demands particular patterns of behaviour. So, for example, if I want to be perceived as masculine and I believe that heavy drinking is part of hegemonic masculinity, then I will be more likely to value and engage in heavy drinking.

The social behaviours that are evaluated as masculine or non-masculine include behaviours for which there are clear gender stereotypes, such as paid work or domestic labour, but they also include health-related behaviours. Courtenay's theory of gender and health (outlined in Chapter 1) defines the importance of health behaviours such as binge drinking to hegemonic masculinity:

> ... health-related beliefs and behaviours, like other social practices that men and women engage in, are a means for demonstrating femininities and masculinities. (Courtenay, 2000, p.1385)

Indeed, health-related behaviours are an important domain for the display of different gender identities (Wearing et al., 1994; Michell & Amos, 1997; de Visser & Smith, 2007a). The importance of health behaviour to gender identity has been highlighted in writing that describes how health behaviours such as binge drinking can be used to reinforce gender stereotypes or resist them (Wood, 2003; Hutton, 2004; de Visser & Smith, 2006, 2007a). For example, in a study of drinking among young men in London (Harnett et al., 2000, p.71), participants noted that 'you've got to be a lad' (p.71), and emphasised the importance of 'keeping pace' with their peers when drinking. As indicated earlier, whether or not a man engages in binge drinking may have implications for his masculine identity. As a result, young men's definitions of drinking as masculine, and the importance to them of being considered to be masculine, may influence their drinking behaviour.

The links between gender and binge drinking may be particularly salient during late adolescence and early adulthood. At this age people have some freedom to explore identities and behaviours without having to commit to them (Erikson, 1968; Arnett, 2000). From this perspective, risky behaviours such as binge drinking are a developmentally appropriate part of young people's identity explorations (Arnett, 2000; Dworkin, 2005; McCreanor et al., 2005). In addition, drinking may be part of young men's socialisation into the adult world (Pape & Hammer, 1996). This highlights the potential importance of binge drinking to the developing gender identities of young men.

## Recent qualitative research

A major focus of the research I have conducted in recent years with Jonathan Smith has been how men's beliefs about masculinity influence their health-related behaviour. Rather than assuming that masculinity is bad for men's health, this research sought to examine more closely the links between masculinity and health-related behaviour. One key focus was how young men can forge a masculine identity that does not involve unhealthy behaviours such as binge drinking.

The research focus was young men's own experiences of growing up, socialising and developing a masculine identity. To allow an examination of young men's experiences, we conducted a qualitative study of 18- to 21-year-old men living in inner London. The sample included two levels of class/socioeconomic opportunity: some men were contacted from job centres and newspaper advertisements, while others were recruited at universities. The sample was also selected to ensure sufficient numbers of white, black and Asian young men. We conducted in-depth interviews with 31 young men to focus on personal experiences of how development of a masculine identity is linked to healthy behaviours such as sport and exercise or unhealthy behaviours such as binge drinking. We also conducted five group discussions involving 27 men to address questions like: How do young men define masculinity? How do they define health? Which behaviours are considered to be healthy or unhealthy? Which behaviours are considered to be masculine or non-masculine? This approach gave an insight into the different ideas about masculinity available in British society, the range of ways of 'being' masculine, and the extent to which different ways of being masculine were deemed acceptable and appropriate.

## Masculinity and alcohol

Men's beliefs about the links between masculinity and drinking were a strong influence on their drinking behaviour. Three broad patterns of association were found, and each will be described in turn.

**Charles**: Some of them, like, they'll just . . . have a drink just to show that they've got bigger balls.

As indicated in the quote above, some men made clear links between masculinity and alcohol consumption: Charles made an association between masculinity, alcohol use, and sexual potency. These men believed that it is important for men to drink, but not only should they drink, they should drink in particular ways. So, men should be able to hold large quantities of alcohol, lest they be labelled a 'lightweight', and they should drink certain forms of alcohol, with beer seen to be more masculine than wine or champagne. For these men, it was clear that if they wanted to be seen as masculine (and view themselves as masculine) they have to be competent drinkers.

A second group of men generally agreed with the first group that drinking is a masculine behaviour. However, these men noted that it is possible to trade 'masculine' competence in one domain for 'non-masculine' behaviour in other domains. For example, participants noted that although Rugby Union star Jonny Wilkinson might be deemed less masculine because he does not drink alcohol, the fact that he had helped England win the World Cup meant that his masculinity was not in question:

**Will**: But do you think Jonny Wilkinson is any less of a man because he doesn't drink? I mean, he's a national hero!

Similarly, some study participants noted that the fact that they were good athletes meant that they could still be regarded as masculine despite not drinking excessively, or abstaining from alcohol:

**Rahul**: . . . because I was better than most of the players, they didn't, like, pressure me into drinking [. . .] that was, that's personally me, but then I have friends who . . . weren't quite as experienced as me at hockey, but just to kind of get into the group I think they felt the need to partake in that.

However, the worrying flipside of the ability to trade masculine competence was that men who feel inadequate in one or more 'masculine' domain may try to make up for this by gaining credit through drinking excessively. For example, quantitative research indicates that problematic alcohol use is more common among men who experience more masculine gender role stress (McCreary et al., 1999). This clearly has implications for health promotion: it suggests that we need to encourage men to develop their masculine identities, and display their masculinity, via behaviours that do not endanger their health.

A third group of men, unlike men in the two groups described above, denied any link between masculinity and alcohol consumption. These men instead valued alternative masculine characteristics. For them, an important marker of masculinity was being independent rather than succumbing to pressure to drink from wider society or from their peers:

**Emeka**: I don't drink, and I feel as masculine as the next guy who does. I feel even more masculine, because I feel that I'm not succumbing to pressure.

These men had strong masculine identities, but they valued 'masculine' characteristics such as rationality and integrity, and some of them even stated that they felt *more* masculine than other men because they were non-drinkers. Some men in this group indicated that their religious beliefs influenced their decision not to drink and their questioning of any links between masculinity and drinking. This was particularly notable for the Muslim men in the study. It is important to note, however, that it was not only the religious young men who questioned links between masculinity and drinking. The existence of this third group shows that it is possible for men to have strong masculine identities that do not involve unhealthy patterns of drinking.

The findings from this study were similar to some of the findings of other recent studies of masculinity and young men's alcohol consumption (Harnett et al., 2000; Mullen et al., 2007). For example, Harnett et al. (2000) found a great diversity in the drinking styles of young men living in London. Diversity in drinking styles was also apparent in a study of young men living in Glasgow (Mullen et al., 2007), which led the authors to suggest that there are not simple links between masculinity and alcohol consumption:

> ... masculinity and drinking [. . .] is less under the sway of hegemonic masculinity and demonstrates more flexibility of role possibilities, with pluralistic masculinities being in operation. We found that young men cannot be treated as a single homogeneous group. (Mullen et al., 2007, p.162)

It is not maleness *per se* – or even masculinity *per se* – that affects binge drinking (Huselid & Cooper, 1992; McCreary et al., 1999; Ricciardelli et al., 2001; Williams & Ricciardelli, 2003; Nolen-Hoeksema, 2004; van Gundy et al., 2005). Instead, binge drinking is an aspect of the embodiment of particular ways of being masculine, and there is not a simple link between masculinity and binge drinking.

### Young men's ambivalence toward alcohol

Previous research into attitudes toward alcohol has revealed that rather than simply having motives for or against drinking, or favourable or unfavourable expectancies for alcohol consumption, most people are ambivalent about alcohol; they perceive compelling reasons to drink and not to drink (Leigh, 1995; Conner & Sparks, 2002; Graham, 2003). This ambivalence is perhaps not surprising given the paradoxical effects of alcohol: it can produce positive *or* negative effects at different stages of a single drinking episode. The existence of such ambivalence is important because if people have both negative and positive evaluations of alcohol, it is more difficult to encourage them to drink less than if they *only* have negative evaluations of alcohol (Armitage, 2003; Conner et al., 2003). It is therefore important to identify aspects of alcohol consumption about which young men are not ambivalent.

Analysis of the data from the study referred to in the previous section revealed that ambivalence toward alcohol is widespread. None of the young male drinkers had uncomplicated positive evaluations of drinking; indeed, all mentioned compelling reasons not to binge drink:

**Daniel**: You wake up in the morning with a hangover . . . with no money. There's loads of downsides. There's more downsides than ups . . . So, when you think of it, why do people drink?

Most motives for drinking were also identified as reasons for not drinking if consumption became excessive; for example, drinking to forget about your worries was good in the short term, but not good if it became excessive:

**Neil**: If you, if you kind of looked at it logically, there shouldn't be a reason why it makes you have a good time, because it's a depressant, and it . . . impairs your ability to do stuff, you know. But for some reason that's fun.

However, three of the reasons given for not drinking were not also motives for drinking: being a victim or perpetrator of violence, the risk of alcoholism, and the financial cost of drinking. These findings suggest that it may be productive to heighten men's concerns about alcohol-related violence and antisocial behaviour, and/or highlight the risks of alcoholism. However, the most promising approach may be to focus on financial disincentives:

**Tim**: . . . we just try to find places that are doing cheap deals that night so that we can actually have a long night where most people would get quite drunk.

Alcohol consumption is 'price elastic': consumption falls when prices rise, and young men's alcohol consumption is particularly price sensitive because their financial resources are more limited. These three unambiguously negative aspects of drinking should be a focus for interventions.

Young men are aware of the downside of drinking – particularly binge drinking – but they also perceive many compelling reasons to drink, including the importance of drinking as an expression of masculine identity. It was noted earlier that there are not simple links between masculinity and binge drinking: young men's ambivalence toward alcohol may also influence their drinking behaviour. It is important, therefore, to work with (or around) young men's ambivalence toward alcohol and focus on reasons for not drinking that men acknowledge as exerting an important influence on their drinking behaviour.

## Quantitative analysis: beliefs and behaviour

Following on from the qualitative research reported in the two preceding sections, I have recently conducted a pilot study to investigate the links between masculinity and alcohol consumption. Questionnaires were completed by 101 university students aged 18–21. The questionnaire assessed different beliefs about masculinity and measured a range of health-related behaviours. The definition of binge drinking used was >8 units of alcohol in one day. This matches the Office of National Statistics definition of 'heavy drinking', and the Prime Minster's Strategy Unit's definition of binge drinking (PMSU, 2004).

Nearly all men (93%) had ever drunk alcohol and 87% had done so in the month prior to completing the questionnaire. Among men who drank any alcohol in the last month, 73% engaged in binge drinking in the last month and 52% engaged in binge drinking in the last week. Within the 52% of men who reported binge drinking in the last week, 22% consumed all of their weekly alcohol intake in binge drinking sessions (i.e. all of their alcohol was consumed on days when they had more than 8 units of alcohol), and 84% consumed more than half of their weekly alcohol in binge-drinking sessions. These data indicate that binge drinking is the most common form of alcohol consumption for these young men.

Masculinity and the links between masculinity and alcohol were assessed using several measures. Gender role conflict (O'Neil et al., 1986) was assessed on four subscales: success, power, competition ('competition': $\alpha$ = .77); restricted emotionality ('restricted emotions': $\alpha$ = .88); restrictive affection between men ('homophobia': $\alpha$ = .87); and conflict between work and family relations ('goal conflict': $\alpha$ = .80). These widely used scales measured general beliefs about male gender roles without specific reference to alcohol consumption.

Three measures of beliefs about masculinity and alcohol consumption were developed for this study. Men also expressed their degree of agreement with the statements that compared to other men 'men who drink are less masculine' and 'men who cannot hold their drink are less masculine'. The third measure of masculinity–alcohol beliefs was constructed from responses to eight items. Men used a 5-point scale to rate the masculinity of eight men, who presented different combinations of three key characteristics of stereotypical hegemonic masculinity: alcohol consumption, football ability and heterosexuality. The data in Figure 6.2 show that, overall, drinkers were rated as more masculine than men who did not drink (black bars: drinkers' mean = 2.9, non-drinkers' mean = 2.7; $t_{(100)}$ = 4.79,

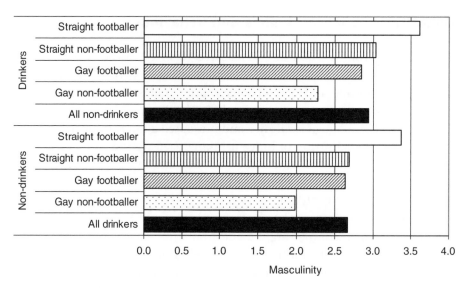

**Figure 6.2** Perceived masculinity of drinkers (top half) and abstainers (bottom half) in a sample of English university students.

$p < .01$). Paired comparisons revealed that, for each of the four groups, men who drank alcohol were deemed to be significantly more masculine than non-drinkers (all significant at $p < .01$) by an average of 0.3 points on the 5-point scale of masculinity.

Data from three measures of attitudes indicate that men who believe that drinking is an important element of masculinity are more likely to binge drink. The overall difference score between the two black bars in Figure 6.2 (drinkers compared to abstainers) was related to binge drinking, such that men who rated drinkers as more masculine reported more binge drinking in the last week ($r = .26$, $p = .01$). Furthermore, less agreement with the statement 'Men who drink are less masculine' was significantly related to more frequent binge drinking in the last week ($r = -.28$, $p < .01$). However, agreement with the statement 'Men who cannot hold their drink are less masculine' was not significantly related to more frequent binge drinking in the last week ($r = .16$, $p = .12$).

There were less clear associations between binge drinking in the last week and scores on subscales of the 'gender role conflict' scale. Binge drinking was significantly related to lower scores on the 'homophobia' ($r = -.21$, $p = .03$) and 'goal conflict' scales ($r = -.23$, $p = .02$), but was not significant related to 'competition' ($r = -.13$, $p = .20$) or 'restricted emotions' ($r = -.06$, $p = .56$). Men who expressed more goal conflict were less likely to binge drink; this may be due to difficulties accommodating binge drinking with a busy work or study schedule. The association between binge drinking and less homophobic attitudes is less easy to explain, and runs counter to expectations that traditional masculine beliefs would be related to more binge drinking (see Huselid & Cooper, 1992; McCreary et al., 1999; Ricciardelli et al., 2001; Williams & Ricciardelli, 2003; Nolen-Hoeksema, 2004; van Gundy et al., 2005).

## Conclusion

Young men are more likely than other members of the population to binge drink. Youth appears to be an important influence on binge drinking, because binge drinking is more common among younger women then older women. However, in addition to youth, 'maleness' or masculinity is an important influence on binge drinking. Previous survey-based research has indicated that perceived heightened masculinity is related to more binge drinking (Huselid & Cooper, 1992; McCreary et al., 1999; Ricciardelli et al., 2001; Williams & Ricciardelli, 2003; Nolen-Hoeksema, 2004; van Gundy et al., 2005). However, it is important to note that such data measure the association between hegemonic or traditional masculinity and binge drinking. Given the widespread acknowledgement that a range of alternative masculinities exist alongside the hegemonic mode (Connell, 1995; Edley & Wetherell, 1999; Frosh et al., 2002), it is important to identify which aspects of masculinity explain young men's heightened propensity for binge drinking.

The qualitative data summarised above indicate that less important than masculinity *per se* are specific beliefs about masculinity and alcohol use. Although many men perceived a link between masculinity and alcohol consumption (and behaved accordingly), other men rejected the notion that binge drinking is an important masculine behaviour (de Visser & Smith, 2007a). These men were able to have strong masculine identities that did not involve excessive alcohol consumption (see also Mullen et al., 2007). The data presented above also revealed widespread ambivalence toward alcohol among young men who binge drink (de Visser & Smith, 2007b). The new quantitative data reported here were collected to examine further the need for specific measures of masculinity and alcohol, rather than general measures of beliefs about masculinity. As expected, it was found that specific measures of beliefs about masculinity and alcohol consumption were stronger correlates of young men's binge drinking than were more general measures of gender role attitudes.

There is a need, therefore, to critique the perceived relationship between masculinity and alcohol consumption and encourage men to develop healthy expressions of masculine identity. Masculinity is multifaceted, rather than unitary: it can be defined and enacted in different ways, and is not necessarily linked to unhealthy behaviours. Indeed, it is possible to draw an analogy between masculinity and alcohol. Used in particular ways, alcohol has some health benefits (White, 1999); used inappropriately or excessively, it has detrimental effects on individual health and social wellbeing (Rehm et al., 2001; PMSU, 2004). Similarly, it is *how* young men define and use their masculinity, rather than how masculine they feel, that determines whether it will harm or benefit their health. The challenge for alcohol harm reduction strategies is to help men to develop masculine identities that do not entail behaviours such as excessive alcohol consumption.

## Acknowledgements

This study was funded by a Sidney Sax Public Health Post-Doctoral Research Fellowship from the Australian National Health and Medical Research Council (Grant 187027) to Richard de Visser. Funding for research costs in London was provided by the United Kingdom Economic and Social Research Council (Grant RES-000-22-0406). Some of the qualitative research presented in this chapter has previously been published elsewhere (de Visser & Smith, 2007a, b).

## References

Andersson, B., Hibell, B., Beck, F. et al. (2007) *Alcohol and Drug Use Among European 17-18 Year Old Students*. Stockholm: Swedish Council for Information on Alcohol and Other Drugs.

Armitage, C. (2003) Beyond attitudinal ambivalence: effects of belief homogeneity on attitude-intention-behaviour relations. *European Journal of Social Psychology*, **33**, 551–563.

Arnett, J. (2000) Emerging adulthood: a theory of development from the late teens through the twenties. *American Psychologist*, **55**, 469–480.

Best, D., Rawaf, S., Rowley, J., Floyd, K., Manning, V. & Strang, J. (2001) Ethnic and gender differences in drinking and smoking among London adolescents. *Ethnicity & Health*, **6**, 51–57.

Borjesson, W. & Dunne, M. (2001) Alcohol expectancies of women and men in relation to alcohol use and perceptions of the effects of alcohol on the opposite sex. *Addictive Behaviours*, **26**, 707–719.

Caspi, A., Begg, D., Dickson, N. et al. (1997) Personality differences predict health-risk behaviours in young adulthood. *Journal of Personality and Social Psychology*, **73**, 1052–1063.

Casswell, S., Pledger, M. & Hooper, R. (2003) Socioeconomic status and drinking patterns in young adults. *Addiction*, **98**, 601–610.

Claussen, B. (1999) Alcohol disorders and re-employment in a 5-year follow-up of long-term unemployed. *Addiction*, **94**, 133–138.

Cochran, S., Keenan, C., Schober, C. & Mays, V. (2000) Estimates of alcohol use and clinical treatment needs among homosexually active men and women in the US population. *Journal of Consulting and Clinical Psychology*, **68**, 1062–1071.

Connell, R. (1987) *Gender & Power*. Cambridge: Polity Press.

Connell, R. (1995) *Masculinities*. Sydney: Allen & Unwin.

Conner, M. & Sparks, P. (2002) Ambivalence and attitudes. *European Review of Social Psychology*, **12**, 37–70.

Conner, M., Povey, R., Sparks, P., James, R. & Shepherd, R. (2003) Moderating role of attitudinal ambivalence within the theory of planned behaviour. *British Journal of Social Psychology*, **42**, 75–94.

Courtenay, W. (2000) Constructions of masculinity and their influence on men's well-being: a theory of gender and health. *Social Science & Medicine*, **50**, 1385–1401.

Day, K., Gough, B. & McFadden, M. (2004) Warning! Alcohol can seriously damage your feminine health: a discourse analysis of recent British newspaper coverage of women and drinking. *Feminist Media Studies*, **4**, 165–185.

Department of Health (2007) *Safe. Sensible. Social. The Next Steps in the National Alcohol Strategy*. London: Department of Health.

Droomers, M., Schrijvers, C., Stronks, K., van de Mheen, D. & Mackenbach, J. (1999) Educational differences in excessive alcohol consumption: the role of psychosocial and material stressors. *Preventive Medicine*, **29**, 1–10.

Dworkin, J. (2005) Risk taking as developmentally appropriate experimentation for college students. *Journal of Adolescent Research*, **20**, 219–241.

Edley, N. & Wetherell, M. (1997) Jockeying for position: the construction of masculine identities. *Discourse and Society*, **8**, 203–217.

Erikson, E. (1968) *Identity: Youth and Crisis*. New York: Norton.

Frosh, S., Phoenix, A. & Pattman, R. (2002) *Young Masculinities*. Basingstoke, UK: Palgrave Macmillan.

Graham, K. (2003) The yin and yang of alcohol intoxication: implications for research on the social consequences of drinking. *Addiction*, **98**, 1021–1023.

van Gundy, K., Schiemean, S., Kelley, M. & Rebellon, C. (2005) Gender role orientations and alcohol use among Moscow and Toronto adults. *Social Science & Medicine*, **61**, 2317–2330.

Hammersley, R. & Ditton, J. (2005) Binge or bout? Quantity and rate of drinking by young people in the evening in licensed premises. *Drugs: Education, Prevention & Policy*, **12**, 493–500.

Hanson, M.D. & Chen, E. (2007) Socioeconomic status and substance use behaviours in adolescents. *Journal of Health Psychology*, **12**, 32–35.

Harnett, R., Thom, B., Herring, R. & Kelly, M. (2000) Alcohol in transition: towards a model of young men's drinking styles. *Journal of Youth Studies*, **3**, 61–77.

Harré, R. & van Langenhove, L. (1998) *Positioning Theory*. Oxford: Blackwell.

Heim, D., Hunter, S., Ross, A. et al. (2004) Alcohol consumption, perceptions of community responses and attitudes to service provision: results from a survey of Indian, Chinese and Pakistani young people in greater Glasgow, Scotland, UK. *Alcohol & Alcoholism*, **39**, 220–226.

Henson, J., Carey, M., Carey, K. & Maisto, S. (2006) Associations among health behaviours and time perspective in young adults: model testing with boot-strapping replication. *Journal of Behavioral Medicine*, **29**, 127–137.

Huselid, R. & Cooper, M. (1992) Gender roles as mediators of sex differences in adolescent alcohol use and abuse. *Journal of Health and Social Behavior*, **33**, 348–362.

Hutton, F. (2004) Up for it, mad for it? Women, drug use and participation in club scenes. *Health, Risk & Society*, **6**, 223–237.

Jackson, C. & Tinkler, P. (2007) 'Ladettes' and 'Modern Girls': 'troublesome' young femininities. *Sociological Review*, **55**, 251–272.

Jefferis, B., Power, C. & Manor, O. (2005) Adolescent drinking level and adult binge drinking in a national birth cohort. *Addiction*, **100**, 543–549.

Johnston, K. & White, K. (2003) Binge-drinking: a test of the role of group norms in the Theory of Planned Behaviour. *Psychology & Health*, **18**, 63–77.

Kimmel, M. & Messner, M. (2003) *Men's Lives*. 6th edn. Boston, MA: Allyn & Bacon.

Kuntsche, E., Rehm, J. & Gmel, G. (2004) Characteristics of binge drinkers in Europe. *Social Science & Medicine*, **59**, 113–127.

Lader, D. & Goddard, E. (2006) *Drinking: Adults' Behaviour and Knowledge in 2006*. London: Office for National Statistics.

Leigh, B. (1995) A thing so fallen, and so vile: images of drinking and sexuality in women. *Contemporary Drug Problems*, **22**, 415–434.

Lemle, R. & Mishkind, M. (1989) Alcohol and masculinity. *Journal of Substance Abuse Treatment*, **6**, 213–222.

Lyons, A., Dalton, S. & Hoy, A. (2006) Hardcore drinking: portrayals of alcohol consumption in young women's and men's magazines. *Journal of Health Psychology*, **11**, 223–232.

Mahalik, J., Lagan, H. & Morrison, J. (2006) Health behaviours and masculinity in Kenyan and US male college students. *Psychology of Men & Masculinity*, **7**, 191–202.

McCarthy, D., Aarons, G. & Brown, S. (2002) Educational and occupational attainment and drinking: an expectancy model in young adulthood. *Addiction*, **97**, 717–726.

McCreanor, T., Greenaway, A., Barnes, H., Borell, S. & Gregory, A. (2005) Youth identity formation and contemporary alcohol marketing. *Critical Public Health*, **15**, 251–262.

McCreary, D.R., Newcomb, M.D. & Sadava, S.W. (1999) The male role, alcohol use, and alcohol problems: a structural equation modelling examination in adult men and women. *Journal of Counseling Psychology*, **46**(1), 109–124.

McQueen, C. & Henwood, K. (2002) Young men in 'crisis': attending to the language of teenage boys' distress. *Social Science & Medicine*, **55**, 1493–1509.

Michell, L. & Amos, A. (1997) Girls, pecking order and smoking. *Social Science & Medicine*, **44**, 1861–1869.

Ministry of Health (2007) *Alcohol Use in New Zealand: Analysis of the 2004 New Zealand Health Behaviours Survey*. Wellington, New Zealand: Ministry of Health.

Montemurro, B. & McClure, B. (2005) Changing gender norms for alcohol consumption: social drinking and lowered inhibitions at bachelorette parties. *Sex Roles*, **52**, 279–288.

Mullen, K., Watson, J., Swift, J. & Black, D. (2007) Young men, masculinity and alcohol. *Drugs: Education, Prevention & Policy*, **14**, 151–165.

Muthén, B. & Muthén, L. (2000) The development of heavy drinking and alcohol-related problems from ages 18 to 37 in a US national sample. *Journal of Studies on Alcohol*, **61**, 290–300.

Nolen-Hoeksema, S. (2004) Gender differences in risk factors and consequences for alcohol use and problems. *Clinical Psychology Review*, **24**, 981–1010.

O'Neil, J., Helms, B., Gable, R., David, L. & Wrightsman, L. (1986) Gender-role conflict scale: college men's fear of femininity. *Sex Roles*, **14**, 335–350.

Pape, H. & Hammer, T. (1996) How does young people's alcohol consumption change during the transition to early adulthood? *Addiction*, **91**, 1345–1357.

Perkins, H. (2002) Social norms and the prevention of alcohol misuse in collegiate contexts. *Journal of Studies on Alcohol*, Suppl.14, 164–172.

Plant, M.L., Plant, M.A. & Mason, W. (2002) Drinking, smoking and illicit drug use among British adults: gender differences explored. *Journal of Substance Use*, **7**, 24–33.

Prime Minister's Strategy Unit (2004) *Alcohol Harm Reduction Strategy for England*. London: Strategy Unit.

Pugh, L.A. & Bry, B.H. (2007) The protective effects of ethnic identity for alcohol and marijuana use among Black young adults. *Cultural Diversity & Ethnic Minority Psychology*, **13**, 187–193.

Rauch, S. & Bryant, J. (2000) Gender and context differences in alcohol expectancies. *Journal of Social Psychology*, **140**, 240–253.

Rehm, N., Room, R. & Edwards, G. (2001) *Alcohol in the European Region: Consumption, Harm and Policies*. Geneva: World Health Organization.

Ricciardelli, L., Connor, J., Williams, R. & Young, R. (2001) Gender stereotypes and drinking cognitions as indicators of moderate and high risk drinking among young women and men. *Drug & Alcohol Dependence*, **61**, 129–136.

Schulenberg, J., O'Malley, P.M., Bachman, J.G., Wadsworth, K.N. & Johnston, L.D. (1996) Getting drunk and growing up: trajectories of frequent binge drinking during the transition to young adulthood. *Journal of Studies on Alcohol*, **57**, 289–304.

Spijkerman, R., van den Eijnden, R. Overbeek, G. & Engels, R. (2007) The impact of peer and parental norms and behavior on adolescent drinking: the role of drinker prototypes. *Psychology & Health*, **22**, 7–29.

Stockwell, T., Heale, P., Chikritzhs, T., Dietze, P. & Catalano, P. (2002) How much alcohol is drunk in Australia in excess of the new Australian alcohol guidelines? *Medical Journal of Australia*, **176**, 91–92.

Substance Abuse and Mental Health Services Administration (2004) *Results from the 2003 National Survey on Drug Use and Health: National Findings*. Rockville, MD: Department of Health and Human Services.

de Visser, R. & Smith, J.A. (2006) Mister in between: a case study of masculine identity and health-related behaviour. *Journal of Health Psychology*, **11**, 685–695.

de Visser, R. & Smith, J.A. (2007a) Alcohol consumption and masculine identity among young men. *Psychology & Health*, **22**, 595–614.

de Visser, R. & Smith, J. (2007b) Young men's ambivalence toward alcohol. *Social Science & Medicine*, **64**, 350–362.

de Visser, R., Rissel, C., Smith, A. & Richters, J. (2006) Sociodemographic correlates of smoking, drinking, injecting drug use, and sexual risk behaviour in a representative sample of Australian young people. *International Journal of Behavioral Medicine*, **13**, 153–162.

Wardle, J. & Steptoe, A. (2003) Socioeconomic differences in attitudes and beliefs about healthy lifestyles. *Journal of Epidemiology & Community Health*, **57**, 440–443.

Wearing, B., Wearing, S. & Kelly, K. (1994) Adolescent women, identity and smoking: leisure experience as resistance. *Sociology of Health & Illness*, **16**, 626–643.

Wechsler, H., Lee, J., Kuo, M., Seibring, M., Nelson, T. & Lee, H. (2002) Trends in college binge drinking during a period of increased prevention efforts. *Journal of American College Health*, **50**, 203–217.

White, I. (1999) The level of alcohol consumption at which all-cause mortality is least. *Journal of Clinical Epidemiology*, **52**, 967–975.

Williams, R. & Ricciardelli, L. (2003) Negative perceptions about self-control and identification with gender-role stereotypes related to binge eating, problem drinking, and co-morbidity among adolescents. *Journal of Adolescent Health*, **32**, 66–72.

Wood, R. (2003) The straightedge youth subculture: observations on the complexity of sub-cultural identity. *Journal of Youth Studies*, **6**, 33–52.

# Chapter 7

# MEN'S MENTAL HEALTH

Elianne Riska

## Introduction

Men's health has been left understudied and untheorised in social science research on health. This void is certainly evident in the area of men's mental health. Women have been the focus of mental health research because of their high rates of diagnosed mental disorders and use of psychotropics – drugs that influence the central nervous system. The classics on gender and mental health have tried to grapple with the reason for women's higher rates (Cooperstock, 1971; Chesler, 1989) and so have left men's mental health issues largely unexplored. Recent research has identified this knowledge gap (Busfield, 1996; Brooks, 2001; Kempner, 2006a), but much research about men's mental health has yet to be done from a gender-sensitive perspective. As scholars have noted, men's mental health has not been a topic of major research or clinical interest in its own right, and even studies that have included men have seldom focused on men's gendered experience (Addis & Cohane, 2005, p.634).

This chapter reviews research and theoretical perspectives on men's mental health. The first part of the chapter looks at the origins of sociological research on gender and mental health in the 1970s. It shows that two theoretical traditions in research on men and mental health can be derived from the early women-focused research: the social-causation and the social-constructionist perspectives (Pugliesi, 1992). The social-causation approach is based on the assumption that gender differences in mental health are real and can be explained by uncovering their structural determinants. The explanations draw on sex role theory, and later researchers have applied a gender difference approach. The social-constructionist perspective challenges the validity of the criteria for defining mental health in social epidemiological research and in biomedical knowledge and clinical practice. In this latter research tradition, the focus was on the methodological issues regarding what produces women's higher rates of mental illness, and second, psychiatric treatment as a form of social control of women. Men's mental health issues were thereby rendered invisible.

This chapter suggests that a gender-sensitive perspective on men's mental health implies that research has to link masculinity and gendered values to definitions and categories of mental disorders. A closer look at men's mental health problems suggests that existing medical categories entail notions of failed masculinity set within a certain historic, economic and social context. Recent post-structuralist theorising on gender and health has analysed men's mental health issues as part of gender performance and the fulfilment of expected gendered cultural scripts. The second part of the chapter will take a closer look at the medicalisation of 'failed' masculinity, especially the medicalisation of certain aspects of middle-class male behaviour. Type A personality, attention deficit and hyperactivity disorder (ADHD) and post-traumatic-stress disorder (PTSD) constitute three examples of medicalised masculinities that point to the link between medical treatments of male mood disorders, social control and men's location in the gender order.

## Rates of mental disorders

Epidemiological research from most western countries shows that women more often than men report mental health disorders. For example, generalised anxiety and depression are reported two to three times as often by women as by men (Pugliesi, 1992; Rieker & Bird, 2000; Courtenay, 2000; Brooks, 2001; Horwitz, 2002; Silverstein, 2002). Women also report use of medications that alleviate such symptoms (e.g. tranquillisers, hypnotics and antidepressants) almost twice as often as men (Ettorre & Riska, 1995; Horwitz & Wakefield, 2007).

Men's lower rates of reported mental illness have been given a number of explanations that follow indirectly from the key efforts to explain women's high rates. The major theoretical framework has been sex role theory. The assumption has been that the adoption of a sex role identity through socialisation makes men's behaviour, unlike women's, incompatible with the adoption of a sick role (Nathanson, 1975; Gerhardt, 1989, p.280). This is the classic 'women-are-expressive' hypothesis that suggests that only women are allowed to experience symptoms, to report them and to seek care (Phillips & Segal, 1969; Cooperstock, 1971; Gove & Tudor, 1973). By contrast, the values of masculinity are assumed to be in conflict with expressing emotions and help-seeking, and men are assumed to channel their emotional expression in different ways. This is the blockage release model of men's emotions (Robinson, 2002). It is assumed that normative expectations about men's mastery of their behaviour lead men to block their emotions and that the consequence is a variety of violent behaviour, i.e. self-destructive behaviour (men have a higher suicide rate than women), drinking and violence towards others (women/spouse). These male behaviours are assumed to constitute a repertoire of mental symptomatology that has been interpreted as functional equivalents to women's diagnosed mental disorders.

Another version of this kind of functionalist explanation of gender-specific release patterns is the substitution hypothesis: it is assumed that men use psychotropic drugs less often than women because men self-medicate everyday stresses and anxieties with alcohol. The substitution hypothesis suggests that psychotropic drugs and alcohol are two gender-specific psychoactive substances. For the 1960s, the gendered choices would have been a martini or a Valium (keeping in mind, however, a solid middle-class context). These images suggest that gender-specific norms in society have created two gender-specific coping mechanisms. As discussed in the previous chapter, men have traditionally used alcohol as a relaxing substance, but until recently this substance use has been viewed negatively for women. Men's self-medication is assumed to be related to their need to maintain their autonomy and internal control, in contrast to the external social control and regulation of women's mental health needs by doctors and the healthcare system (Cooperstock, 1971, p.242).

The notion of two gender-segmented, functionally equivalent chemical coping patterns conceals, however, the contextual differences between men's and women's use of substances (Ettorre & Riska, 1995, pp.36–37). While alcohol can be accessed freely and is generally consumed in public and in a social context, psychotropics are prescription drugs and generally consumed in private. Although dependency on both substances has been a matter of public concern, current psychotropic drugs – notably the new generation of antidepressants – are, in contrast to the benzodiazepines of the 1970s and 1980s, claimed to be free from dependency-producing effects.

The foregoing cultural explanation of men's mental health behaviour has been amended with a structural evaluation of the consequences of the sex roles. Still working within the theoretical framework of the sex role theory, the early work in the area interpreted gender differences in mental health as a consequence of the economic and social differences linked to the two gender positions. The health consequences are assumed to be related to two conditions: differential exposure and differential vulnerability related to the gender roles (Rieker & Bird, 2000; Brooks, 2001). The thesis about differential exposure suggests that men are less exposed than women to conflicting expectations and role strain, and men's role accumulation results in mental health advantages for men (Gove & Tudor, 1973, p.814). This model of a universal mental health benefit for men is challenged by the thesis about differential vulnerability. This thesis contextualises the stressors and suggests that the same role demands – family or work – have different meanings for men and women and, furthermore, that moderating factors – coping resources, coping strategies, and social support – have different meanings and implications for men and women (Thoits, 1995).

The differential vulnerability model has been incorporated in more recent gender difference research. In this research the focus is on examining how much 'real' difference remains when the actual social positions of men and women are compared. Depression among men has been the focus of American research, and the impact of changing female roles on men's mental health has been a central theme in the *Journal of Health and Social Behavior* (e.g. Rosenfield, 1992). In contrast to the quantitative approach of American researchers, recent research in the UK on men's depression has used a qualitative approach and analysed men's narrative accounts of their experience of mental health problems and depression in relation to their notions of masculinity (e.g. McQueen & Henwood, 2002; Emslie et al., 2006).

The cultural model – generally referred to as the gender identity model – and the structural model of the social implications of the gender positions on mental health contain at least four weaknesses.

First, the view of men as possessing mental health benefits related to their advantaged social position entails a homogenisation of men. This view results not only in the confirmation of a binary notion of gender but also in a neglect of differences between men, especially in making disadvantaged men invisible.

Second, the view that considers traditional masculinity as lethal for men not only succumbs to the fallacy of homogenising men but leads also to a pathologising of masculinity as a cultural trait. Compulsory traditional masculinity is assumed to be a normative muster requiring conformity and proofs. Hence, upholding the values and behaviours of traditional masculinity is assumed to result in health risks and mental health implications for men (Courtenay, 2000; Lohan, 2007). Far from being historical thinking, the notion of men as the victims of traditional masculinity is an essentialist notion of manhood that has gained new currency in public health thinking about men's physical and mental health (e.g. Harrison et al., 1989; Meryn & Jadad, 2001).

Third, the key efforts to explain women's mental disorders have implied that the conceptual tools for explaining men's social disadvantages and male role stressors are either deficient or nonexistent. The current theoretical frameworks that draw on gender role theory provide only indirect or left-over explanations of men's mental health. This means that whatever condition is not causal for women's mental disorders is the explanatory factor for men's. This kind of argument is not only erroneous but provides deficient analytical tools for explaining men's mental health problems. While social science research seems in general to be characterised by a lack of theorising about men and masculinities (Hearn, 1998), research on mental health is particularly weak in this respect. In mental health research, the theoretical explanations accentuate the absence, avoidance and untheorised presence of men.

Fourth, the use of rates of diagnosed psychiatric pathology or certain indicators of mental symptoms restricts attention to certain gendered responses. An approach that takes as its departure certain categories of mental illness and symptom expressions offers a limited view of men's mental health. By contrast, an approach that looks at the social construction of masculinity and its implications for men's mental wellbeing provides a broader framework for understanding men's mental disorders.

## The social-constructionist perspective

For early psychiatry, manhood was a taken-for-granted category, and men's mental health problems, in contrast to women's, were seldom problematised. As Lunbeck (1998, p.84) notes about the early decades of twentieth-century American psychiatry, 'The models of manliness that psychiatrists put forth . . . were contradictory and largely untheorised, patched together in practice, informed by their own largely unexamined experiences as men.' A critique of the construction of mental health categories and of the gendered character of these categories grew in the latter part of the twentieth century. In the 1960s psychiatry came under heavy attack from critics in the US and the UK, from a group of scholars who have been termed the 'anti-psychiatry movement' (Crossley, 1998; Horwitz 2002, pp.62–63). This was a critique of psychiatry, its knowledge basis, its scientific validity and the efficacy of the suggested treatments – a critique that was largely gender neutral. This movement had, however, gendered implications. In the early 1970s, women's health advocates and feminist scholars turned their gaze toward women's mental health and used the claims of the anti-psychiatry movement. The theme of using medical knowledge and treatments as a way of exerting social control was given a gendered content: medicine maintained women's subordination in society. A classic was Chesler's (1972/1989) *Women and Madness*. Despite its title, it included an analysis of men's mental health. Chesler argued that men were constructed as the standard for rational behaviour and mental health against which women's behaviours were evaluated. Empirical studies showed that the standard of generic mental health was unconditionally attributed to fit the behaviour and mood of men but not women (Chesler, 1989; Busfield, 1996). As Pugliesi (1992, p.60) in her analysis of research traditions about gender and mental health notes, 'The social structures of gender, conceptions of mental health and epidemiological practice interact to construct what appear to be "objective" differences in the mental health of women and men.'

Men's advantaged position in society or, in today's terminology, the hegemony of men (Hearn, 2004) maintained women as the primary target in the definition of mental disorders. It was not only feminists who criticised the sexism inherent in psychiatric practice. The scholarly community also pointed out the gender bias of the theory and practice of psychiatry, a claim presented by Dohrenwend and Dohrenwend (1976, p.1451) in a classic article in which they suggested that women's higher rates of mental illness was a matter of the social construction of illness categories. They argued that the explanation for gender differences in mental health is methodological rather than substantive. In their words, 'It seems plausible . . . to interpret these results as being a function of changes in concepts and methods for defining what constitutes a psychiatric case' (Dohrenwend & Dohrenwend, 1976, p.1452). In reviewing studies about gender and mental disorders, Dohrenwend and Dohrenwend found that studies before 1950 in the US largely reported a higher incidence of psychiatric disorders among men than among women, while studies after 1950 reported the reverse. According to them, the studies before 1950 used data given by officials who tended to report personality disorders and schizophrenia common among men and were less likely to provide information about neurotic symptoms common among women because of these symptoms' private character. By contrast, studies after 1950 used respondents' self-reported symptoms, and the battery of questions about symptoms focused on anxiety and depression and therefore mapped the territory of women's symptomatology while overlooking men's repertoire of more aggressive symptoms (Dohrenwend & Dohrenwend, 1976, p.1452). As later observers on gendered notions of mental health have noted, men's emotional reactions, substance abuse and violence are not subject to psychiatric interpretation, because 'male disorders do not harbor the implication of mental disorderedness or weakness to the same degree as female disorders such as depression or PMS' (Pugliesi, 1992, p.62).

The social-constructionist approach to mental health derives from the labelling approach to deviance and that approach's descendant, the medicalisation thesis. That thesis was introduced by Irving Zola (1972) to serve as a conceptual tool in understanding the increasing influence and implication of medicine as a broad culture and cadre of expertise. It came to be used as a theoretical framework for understanding the role of medicine as a mechanism of social control, especially of the socially disadvantaged by gender, race and ethnicity. The theme of medicalisation suggested that medicine was a surveillance technology to control deviance embodied by disadvantaged groups. Some feminist writers used medicalisation as an analytical framework to highlight the pathologisation of women's body, symptoms and cultural traits. The focus on the social construction of medicalised categories of mental illness for women turned attention away from illuminating how men's mental symptomatology was constructed. The female gendering of the medicalisation thesis rendered invisible the processes that medicalised men's mental health (Riska, 2003, 2004; Rosenfeld & Faircloth, 2006; Conrad 2007). Two recent areas of research can serve here as examples of the social construction of maleness and mental disorders. The first area is the construction of patienthood in advertising for psychotropic drugs and the second is the construction of categories of medicalised masculinities such as Type A, ADHD, and the post-combat disorders called post-traumatic stress disorder (PTSD) and Gulf War syndrome (GWS).

## Gender portrayals in advertising of psychotropic drugs

Psychotropic drugs influence the central nervous system and are prescribed for mood disorders. There are four categories of such drugs: antipsychotics, antidepressants, tranquillisers and hypnotics. During the past 30 years, each decade has been characterised by a belief that a new drug category is a panacea. The 1960s witnessed the increasing sales of antipsychotics and debated their correct dosage and their side effects. The 1970s and 1980s – the age of Valium and Halcion – were characterised by a concern over the widespread use and the dependency produced by a long-term use of tranquillisers and hypnotics, especially those based on benzodiazepines (Speaker, 1997). The 1990s and after – the antidepressant era – have been characterised by the rising sales of the new generation of antidepressants called SSRIs (selective serotonin-reuptake inhibitors) (Healy, 1997, 2004).

Studies of the use of psychotropic drugs in western countries have consistently reported a higher rate of use among women (Cooperstock, 1971; Ettorre & Riska, 1995; Horwitz & Wakefield, 2007). If men appeared in the reporting on use, they were often there as a mere dummy variable so as to highlight women's high use. The early debate about the medically valid use of psychotropic drugs focused on women's high use, which in the age of tranquillisers and hypnotics was largely a criticism of the dependency-producing effects of these drugs. Men's lower level of use was largely treated as unproblematic, because it either was considered a 'correct' level (e.g. in the use of antipsychotics for schizophrenia) or else a product of the underdiagnosis of men's mental symptoms. A number of studies also referred to the substitution hypothesis – men using alcohol instead – and took this thesis as a verified fact. But as an explanation for men's lower use of tranquillisers or antidepressants, the widely cited substitution hypothesis is a mere assumption that has never been put to empirical test.

Apart from the epidemiology-based studies of gender differences in the use of psychotropic drugs, studies on advertising for psychotropic drugs constitute another genre of research. A large proportion of these studies were completed during the era before direct advertising to patients was allowed. Pharmaceutical companies had therefore to influence the physicians' prescribing habits and convince physicians not only of the need for prescribing a psychotropic drug but also for prescribing a certain brand. General anxiety is a broad category of diffuse symptoms, and the discursive approach of advertisements was to convince doctors that certain mental symptoms needed a certain medication. Research about this has been mostly American. The American advertising for psychotropic drugs showed that by gendering patienthood and by gendering specific drugs, a gender-segmented market could be created (Leppard et al., 1993; Lupton, 1993). A majority of the advertisements for psychotropic drugs and the most gender-stereotypical ones portrayed women.

In these American studies at the time (largely from the mid-1970s to the late 1980s) there was hardly any interest in analysing the advertisements portraying male users. The American trend of women's predominance in the portrayal of users of psychotropic drugs was upheld as a 'universal' finding. This American pattern was not reflected in a series of studies of the gender of portrayed psychotropic drug users in Scandinavian medical advertising. For example, a study of the advertisements for psychotropic drugs that appeared in Scandinavian medical journals in 1975, 1985 and 1995 showed that, contrary to the results of the American studies, men were in the majority of the user pictures in 1975 (Lövdahl & Riska, 2000).

The male majority derived from the dominance of advertisements for antipsychotic drugs, and the gender portrayals in the advertising for this drug category confirmed the gendered character of patienthood for this drug.

Advertising for tranquillisers and hypnotics dominated the advertising for psychotropic drugs in western countries in 1985, but again the gender portrayals in Scandinavian advertising differed from the American ads. American studies tended to show the need for these drugs to be based in women's traditional role as a wife and mother. Although female users were in a majority of the Scandinavian user ads in 1985, both women's and men's need of psychotropic drugs were shown as related to demands at work (Lövdahl & Riska, 2000).

The Prozac era – a metaphor for the marketing and rising consumption of a new generation of antidepressants, SSRIs – has introduced a new discourse in the gendering of mental patienthood and of this group of psychotropics. Both the medical and public discourse of SSRI-type antidepressants tend in the US and Ireland to portray these drugs by female images (Blum & Stracuzzi, 2004; Curry & O'Brien, 2006). Again the portrayal of gender in the advertisements for psychotropics differs in Scandinavia. In Scandinavian medical advertising in 2000, half of the advertisements for antidepressants portray only a male. There were some differences between the Scandinavian journals: half of the advertising for psychotropics in Denmark and a third of the advertisements in Norway and Sweden contained portrayals of male users only (Heikell & Riska, 2004). In the portrayal of Scandinavian men's emotional problems, two discourses appeared. One theme in the pictures of male users was the ability of antidepressants to restore men's ability to bond with family (relaxed and smiling middle-aged men were shown helping their parents or children) and hence to address men's difficulties in establishing emotional relationships – a syndrome that has been presented as the mental cost of 'traditional masculinity'. The other theme was the medication of men's ontological insecurity. In the pictures, such insecurity is visualised by drawings of monsters and devils, representations of men's cosmic despair and their problems of existential survival as men.

Both discourses – men's emotional insufficiency and cosmic despair – have to be viewed within the context of the public policy of gender equality in Scandinavia. First, men are supposed to be involved 'new' fathers. This new cultural representation of fatherhood contains an expectation that men should be involved in caregiving and the nurturing of their children and elderly parents along with their working wife (Holter, 2007). The ads suggest that the cultural expectations and the actual conduct of caregiving men produce anxiety and that some men have trouble in performing the expected emotional labour. Second, suicide rates for men are, as in most western countries, two to three times higher than for women, and this gender health inequality has been pointed out in Scandinavian public health programmes. The advertisements for antidepressants suggest that the medication helps men adapt to the new values and norms of Scandinavian masculinity in the era of gender equality.

While anxiety and depression have increasingly been viewed as gendered symptoms, until recently more mundane mental health problems like headache have largely been unanalysed from a gender perspective. A recent American study of marketing of migraine drugs showed the female gendering of headaches and the product for alleviating the symptoms (Kempner, 2006b). The results suggest that the pharmaceutical industry directs its marketing of migraine drugs to women and thereby excludes men who suffer from the condition and who could benefit from the medication. By contrast, cluster headaches have been constructed as a disorder predominant in men and as a disorder of excess masculinity. When women have been diagnosed with this condition, medical discourse has, for example, constructed the masculine facial features of the female patients as a reason for the disorder (Kempner, 2006a).

## Over- and underachievement as a male mental health syndrome

The origin of the aetiological story about men's stress symptoms and their harmful connection to men's health is an often underreported tale of the social construction of masculinity and health. It all began in the early 1950s, when two American cardiologists, Meyer Friedman and Ray Rosenman, suggested that a certain type of aggressive masculine behaviour predicted men's proneness to heart disease. A new risk factor to men's health – Type A – emerged in medical discourse, and Type A Behavioral Pattern was later constructed as the Type A personality in psychological discourse (Riska, 2004). The proneness to heart disease was assumed to reside in the negative emotions of these men. Hostility, anger and aggression were defined as the gendered health risks of hard work required in entrepreneurial and executive positions in the American business world. It was not failure to conform to the norm of healthy middle-class manhood that was of concern to medicine, but rather over-conformity to traditional masculine behaviour like that of the excessively competitive and hyperactive Type A man. This was the first time that men's competitive and aggressive behaviour was seen in pathological terms rather than as the normal cultural repertoire of masculine behaviour. It was the hypermasculinity of Type A men that was constructed as an emotional health hazard with implications for men's cardiac health. Although the Type A thesis was declared invalid in medicine in the mid 1980s, the thesis about the toxicity of hypermasculinity continued to exist for yet another decade in the US as a form of lay epidemiology.

When adult American men 50 years later began to self-diagnose impulsive and hyperactive behaviour not in terms of deviance but rather as part of a medical syndrome called ADHD, at issue was not a medicalisation of the reasons for overperformance but for underachievement (Conrad, 2007, pp.49–60). As scholars have pointed out, ADHD is a profoundly gendered phenomenon: it is primarily a medicalisation of boys' inability to succeed in the educational system (Hart et al., 2006, p.134). ADHD is largely a middle-class definition of underachievement and status anxiety among parents who fear that their (male) children will not manage to maintain their class position through the educational system. Ritalin, a powerful amphetamine drug, is used to produce self-discipline and emotional control among boys who are seen, especially in the institutional context of kindergarten and school, as too impulsive and hyperactive. While ADHD was a condition that from the 1960s to the 1980s concerned boys, in the 1990s adult men began to see ADHD as a medical condition that had not been 'correctly' diagnosed in their childhood. Since the 1990s both professional and lay media have covered the prevalence of adult ADHD. As Conrad (2007, p.64) suggests, the adult ADHD diagnosis is constructed as a 'real' learning disability rooted in a biomedical cause.

In conclusion, it is not only women's emotional instability that has been defined as a medical disorder and constructed as a medical category in medical discourse (Chesler, 1989; Busfield, 1996). Men's emotional instability has also been subjected to medical control and linked to their incapacity to pursue the rational, self-disciplined and goal-directed behaviour expected of 'normal' men (Seidler, 2007). Both Type A Behavioral Pattern, later called Type A personality, and 50 years later ADHD deviated from the expected middle-class male mood, because these males were too hyperactive and aggressive and had lost their capacity to focus on the expected goal of material success. Psychiatry constructed these moods and hypermasculinity in its scientific discourse as medical categories. For example, AHDH and even its adult version have found their way into the prevailing disease classificatory system called DSM-IV (Conrad, 2007, p.57).

Type A personality is a case of later demedicalisation, because when the Type A hypothesis began to be empirically tested with larger population samples than middle-class men, for example women and other social classes of men, the constructed medical category could not be empirically verified. Hence, the thesis was declared scientifically invalid and abandoned in the early 1980s (Riska, 2004). By contrast, educational inattention continues to be a medical label offered by doctors. In addition it has also become a self-diagnosis made not only by adult men but also by a new college-aged cohort. The latter group resorts to powerful psychostimulants, like Ritalin or Adderall, to secure their educational achievement (Loe et al., 2006). For these college students, the male-gendered norm of educational achievement has compelled them, regardless of gender, to resort to Ritalin as a medical technology for attaining a medically disciplined body, enhanced for the expected educational achievement.

The two foregoing cases of medicalisation of male-gendered moods and expected goal-directed masculine behaviour represent two phases of medicalisation of masculinity and the concomitant constitution of medical categories. Type A personality represents the classical version of medicalisation (Conrad, 2007), when representatives of the medical profession and later psychologists not only defined and constructed Type A as a medical category but also acted as the primary agents in its later demedicalisation. By contrast, ADHD is a condition that fits the conceptual framework of the biomedicalisation thesis (Clarke et al., 2003). This thesis suggests that the agents of medicalisation have been blurred and that in fact individuals participate in the medicalisation of their own condition as a way of constructing an enhanced version of their self. The biomedicalisation thesis has pointed to the tendency of biomedicine and technoscience to construct a 'natural' and 'real' body. Current medical consumerism and lifestyle medicine offer opportunities to restore the 'natural' body to fit the 'authentic' notion of the self (Pitts-Taylor, 2007; Rose, 2007).

## Men, warfare and mental health

Throughout human history the mental health effects of warfare have been expected to be part of living the life of a normal and healthy man. For men, proving themselves in the battlefield was in the past a rite of passage and proof of entering manhood. Modern medicine instituted a division of labour in treating the physical and psychological wounds that warfare inflicted on men's bodies. While the medical knowledge and techniques of surgery progressed as a side effect of mending mutilated male bodies, psychiatry has had a special task in interpreting men's claims of post-combat ailments and demands for compensation from the larger society and governmental institutions.

Various terms have been introduced in the effort to find an appropriate medical label for war veterans' anxieties and traumas from experiences in combat. During World War I, war syndromes were interpreted within an organic model: the terms 'shell shock', 'conversion hysteria' and 'combat trauma' were used to describe the organic cause of men's psychological breakdown on the battlefield. Later the term 'combat stress reactions' (CSR) was deployed for mental health problems related to functional incapacity in combat (Jones, 2006, p.534). More recently post-traumatic stress disorder (PTSD) was introduced as a medical category and institutionalised in the DSM-III in 1980. PTSD is an umbrella category for a variety of mental health effects following an unusually traumatic event.

The Vietnam War resulted in the application of PTSD as a medical category explaining the post-combat disorders of Vietnam War veterans who wanted treatment and government compensation for their mental health problems. There is a marked difference in the medicalised masculinities that underlie the diagnosis of PTSD of the Vietnam War veterans and the diagnosis of GWS of the Gulf War veterans. The differences in the medicalised masculinities underlying these two diagnoses can only be understood by looking at the changes in the contemporary culture of masculinity in America.

In her study of Vietnam War veterans undergoing therapy, Kratner (1995) traces the claim for medical legitimacy of the mental ailments that these men suffered. The Vietnam War veterans resisted the label of mental illness, which was connected with weakness and femininity. Instead, their symptoms were presented as a situational disorder that had to be seen as extreme forms of masculine behaviour – hypermasculinity – induced under unusual combat conditions. The label PTSD was a medical model of extreme forms of traditional masculine behaviour (anger, aggression, emotional distance) that was viewed as a result of a selective and stress-related effect of combat. For these men, the relocation to civilian life also meant a confrontation with changed gender norms because various social movements of the 1960s and 1970s – anti-war, civil rights and the women's movement – had brought about a cultural feminisation of society. A medicalisation of hypermasculinity became the framework for how their ailments were discursively constructed.

In more recent wars the label of mental illness or stress-related illness has been seen by war veterans as a de-legitimation of the demands for compensation for combat-inflicted physical and psychological injuries. Gulf War syndrome is an example of how the health costs of war came to be attributed to environmental hazards rather than to a stress-related illness. The latter framework focuses on individual psychopathology and minimises the effects of toxic substances and environmental conditions (Brown et al., 2000, p.246). Environmental hazards, related to the toxins involved in biological warfare, have been claimed to have damaged the bodies and central nervous system of the veterans of the Gulf War. The external origin of the causes for the medical legitimation has to be seen against the re-masculinisation taking place in American culture in the 1980s and 1990s, when popular culture presented re-masculinised images of American masculinity (e.g. Rambo, the Terminator). Although GWS is a contested environmental illness (Brown et al., 2000), the external character of toxins relieves war veterans from any label of an internal failed masculinity as the cause of the ailments.

## Conclusion

The early feminist critique (Millman & Kanter, 1975) of knowledge production in sociology suggested that basic theories and methodologies of that discipline had been limited by the particular interests, perspectives and experiences of (white) men. In the field of mental health the general claim of women's invisibility has not been made. Instead, women have been the key focus, and in fact this has resulted in men's mental health problems being neglected and under-theorised. This chapter has reviewed the early mental health research that established the women-focused trend and resulted in a one-dimensional picture of *both* women's and men's mental health concerns. The sex role theory is still the tacit framework for much research on gender differences in mental health although the major focus has shifted to the mediating cultural or material structures that are assumed to explain such differences.

The social-constructionist perspective challenged the validity of the medical categories used in classifying mental health disorders and set the stage for a broader gender analysis of images of mental health and the role of medical experts in defining and confirming categories through treatment practices. Much of this early research was done within the tradition of the medicalisation thesis, which saw the medical profession as the major agent in the social regulation of social behaviour and subordinated social groups. More recently the medical-dominance argument has been supplanted by a theoretical model inspired by the Foucauldian or post-structuralist theorising that points to the blurred boundaries between agency and structure. Accordingly, individuals are not merely docile objects in the labelling of their illness but can also be active participants in constructing the medical legitimation of their medical diagnosis. This process can involve a challenge of the applicability of existing medical categories and presentation of alternative aetiological explanations. Adult ADHD is a case of consumer-driven medical legitimation among adult men who use the medical framework to appeal to organic reasons for a self-perceived underperformance in later life (Conrad, 2007). By contrast, GWS is a case of war veterans attributing their symptoms, including mental disorders, to environmental reasons rather than to individual psychopathology. The environmental aetiological claim relieves these men from doubts about failed masculinity as the underlying reason for their vulnerability to post-combat disorders.

A clearer gender focus on men's mental health and mental disorders is needed in future research in order to promote a broader understanding of different men and masculinities. Such a focus is also needed in order to achieve a theoretical understanding of the complex process in the application and utilisation of new biotechnologies and the individual's search for a more authentic self (Rose, 2007). The cultural appeal of individualism and self-reliance and of repairing and shaping the body and mind for such challenges make men particularly vulnerable to such options because of an identification of masculinity with self-reliance and self-control. Seidler (2007, p.20) urges us therefore to think 'in new ways about transformations of diverse cultural masculinities that can heal unsustainable splits between men's power, bodies, emotions, and pleasures'.

## References

Addis, M.E. & Cohane, G.H. (2005) Social scientific paradigms and their implications for research and practice in men's mental health. *Journal of Clinical Psychology*, **61**(6), 633–647.

Blum, L.M. & Stracuzzi, N.F. (2004) Gender in the Prozac nation: popular discourse and productive femininity. *Gender & Society*, **18**(3), 269–286.

Brooks, G.R. (2001) Masculinity and men's mental health. *Journal of American College Health*, **49**, 285–297.

Brown, P., Zavestoksi, S., McCormick, S., Linder, M., Mandelbaum, J. & Luebke, T. (2000) A gulf of difference: disputes over Gulf War-related illnesses. *Journal of Health and Social Behavior*, **42**(3), 235–257.

Busfield, J. (1996) *Men, Women and Madness: Understanding Gender and Mental Disorder*. London: Macmillan.

Chesler, P. (1989, orig. 1972) *Women and Madness*. New York: Harcourt Brace Jovanovich.

Clarke, A.E., Shim, J.K., Mamo, L., Fosket, J.R. & Fishman, J.R. (2003) Biomedicalization: technoscientific transformations of health and illness, and US biomedicine. *American Sociological Review*, **68**(2), 161–194.

Conrad, P. (2007) *The Medicalization of Society*. Baltimore, MD: Johns Hopkins University Press.

Cooperstock, R. (1971) Sex differences in the use of mood-modifying drugs: an explanatory model. *Journal of Health and Social Behavior*, **12**, 238–244.

Courtenay, W.H. (2000) Constructions of masculinity and their influence on men's well-being: a theory of gender and health. *Social Science and Medicine*, **50**(10), 1385–1401.

Crossley, N. (1998) R.D. Laing and the British anti-psychiatry movement: a socio-historical analysis. *Social Science and Medicine*, **47**(7), 877–889.

Curry, P. & O'Brien, M. (2006) The male heart and the female mind: a study in the gendering of antidepressants and cardiovascular drugs in advertisements in Irish medical publication. *Social Science and Medicine*, **62**(8), 1970–1977.

Dohrenwend, B.P. & Dohrenwend, B.S. (1976) Sex differences and psychiatric disorders. *American Journal of Sociology*, **81**(6), 1447–1454.

Emslie, C., Ridge, D., Ziebland, S. & Hunt, K. (2006) Men's account of depression: reconstructing or resisting hegemonic masculinity? *Social Science and Medicine*, **62**(9), 2246–2257.

Ettorre, E. & Riska, E. (1995) *Gendered Moods: Psychotropics and Society*. London: Routledge.

Gerhardt, U. (1989) *Ideas about Illness: An Intellectual and Political History of Medical Sociology*. Basingstoke, UK: Macmillan.

Gove, W.R. & Tudor, J.F. (1973) Adult sex roles and mental illness. *American Journal of Sociology*, **78**(4), 812–835.

Harrison, J., Chin, J. & Ficarrotto, T. (1989) Warning: masculinity may be dangerous to your health. In: *Men's Lives* (eds M.S. Kimmel & M.A. Messner), pp.246–309. New York: Macmillan.

Hart, N., Grand, N. & Riley, K. (2006) Making the grade: the gender gap, ADHD, and the medicalization of boyhood. In: *Medicalized Masculinities* (eds D. Rosenfeld & C. Faircloth), pp.132–164. Philadelphia, PA: Temple University Press.

Healy, D. (1997) *The Antidepressant Era*. Cambridge, MA: Harvard University Press.

Healy, D. (2004) *Let Them Eat Prozac: The Unhealthy Relationship between the Pharmaceutical Industry and Depression*. New York: New York University Press.

Hearn, J. (1998) Theorizing men and men's theorizing: varieties of discursive practices in men's theorizing of men. *Theory and Society*, **27**(6), 781–816.

Hearn, J. (2004) From hegemonic masculinity to the hegemony of men. *Feminist Theory*, **5**(1), 49–72.

Heikell, T. & Riska, E. (2004) Men's emotional inexpressivity: advertising for psychotropic drugs in Scandinavian journals. *Nordisk Alkohol- och Narkotikatidskrift* (English supplement), **21**, 53–62.

Holter, Ø.G. (2007) Men's work and family reconciliation in Europe. *Men and Masculinities*, **9**(4), 425–456.

Horwitz, A.V. (2002) *Creating Mental Illness*. Chicago, IL: University of Chicago Press.

Horwitz, A.V. & Wakefield, J.C. (2007) *The Loss of Sadness: How Psychiatry Transformed Normal Sorrow into Depressive Disorder*. New York: Oxford University Press.

Jones, E. (2006) Historical approaches to post-combat disorders. *Philosophical Transactions of the Royal Society*, **361**, 533–542.

Kempner, J. (2006a) Uncovering the man in medicine: lessons learned from a study of cluster headache. *Gender and Society*, **20**(5), 632–656.

Kempner, J. (2006b) Gendering the migraine market: do representations of illness matter? *Social Science and Medicine*, **63**(8), 1986–1997.

Kratner, T.X. (1995) Medicalizing masculinity: post traumatic stress disorder in Vietnam veterans. *Masculinities*, **3**(4), 23–65.

Leppard, W., Ogletree, S.M. & Wallen, E. (1993) Gender stereotyping in medical advertising: much ado about something? *Sex Roles*, **29**(11/12), 829–838.

Loe, M.E., DeWitt, C., Quirindongo, C. & Sandler, R. (2006) *'Pharming' to Perform in the Classroom: Making Sense of the Medically-Disciplined College Student Body.* American Sociological Association, Montreal Convention Center, Montreal, Quebec, Canada.

Lohan, M. (2007) How might we understand men's health better? Integrating explanations from critical studies on men and inequalities in health. *Social Science and Medicine*, **65**(3), 493–504.

Lövdahl, U. & Riska, E. (2000) The construction of gender and mental health in Nordic psychotropic-drug advertising. *International Journal of Health Services*, **30**(2), 387–406.

Lunbeck, E. (1998) American psychiatrists and the Modern Man, 1900 to 1920. *Men and Masculinities*, **1**(1), 58–86.

Lupton, D. (1993). The construction of patienthood in medical advertising. *International Journal of Health Services*, **23**(4), 805–819.

McQueen, C. & Henwood, K. (2002) Young men in 'crisis': attending to the language of teenage boys' distress. *Social Science and Medicine*, **55**(9), 1493–1509.

Meryn, S. & Jadad, A.R. (2001) The future of men and their health: are men in danger of extinction? (Editorial). *British Medical Journal*, **323**(1), 1013–1014.

Millman, M. & Kanter, R.M. (1975) Editorial introduction. In: *Another Voice: Feminist Perspectives on Social Life and Social Science* (eds M. Millman & R.M. Kanter), pp. vii–xvii. Garden City, NY: Anchor Press/Doubleday.

Nathanson, C.A. (1975) Illness and the feminine role: a theoretical review. *Social Science and Medicine*, **9**, 57–62.

Phillips, D.L. & Segal, B.E. (1969) Sexual status and psychiatric symptoms. *American Sociological Review*, **34** (February), 58–72.

Pitts-Taylor, V. (2007) *Surgery Junkies: Wellness and Pathology in Cosmetic Culture.* New Brunswick, NJ: Rutgers University Press.

Pugliesi, K. (1992) Women and mental health: two traditions of feminist research. *Women & Health*, **19**(2/3), 43–68.

Rieker, P.R. & Bird, C.E. (2000) Sociological explanations of gender differences in mental and physical health. In: *Handbook of Medical Sociology* (eds C.E. Bird, P. Conrad & A.M. Fremont), pp. 98–113. Upper Saddle River, NJ: Prentice Hall.

Riska, E. (2003) Gendering the medicalization thesis. *Advances in Gender Research: Gender Perspectives on Health and Medicine*, **7**, 59–87.

Riska, E. (2004) *Masculinity and Men's Health: Coronary Heart Disease in Medical and Public Discourse.* Lanham, MD: Rowman & Littlefield.

Robinson, S. (2002) Men's liberation, men's wounds: emotion, sexuality and reconstruction of masculinity in the 1970s. In: *Boys Don't Cry? Rethinking Narratives of Masculinity and Emotion in the US* (eds M. Shamir & J. Travis), pp.205–229. New York: Columbia University Press.

Rose, N. (2007) *The Politics of Life Itself: Biomedicine, Power, and Subjectivity in the Twenty-first Century*. Princeton, NJ: Princeton University Press.

Rosenfeld, D. & Faircloth, C. (2006) *Medicalized Masculinities*. Philadelphia, PA: Temple University Press.

Rosenfield, S. (1992) The cost of sharing: wives' employment and husbands' mental health. *Journal of Health and Social Behavior*, **33**(3), 213–225.

Seidler, V.J. (2007) Masculinities, bodies, and emotional life. *Men and Masculinities*, **10**(1), 9–21.

Silverstein, B. (2002) Gender differences in the prevalence of somatic versus pure depression: a replication. *American Journal of Psychiatry*, **159**(6), 1051–1052.

Speaker, S. (1997) From 'Happiness Pills' to 'National Nightmare': changing cultural assessment of minor tranquilizers in America, 1955–1980. *Journal of the History of Medicine and Allied Sciences*, **52**, 338–376.

Thoits, P.A. (1995) Stress, coping, and social support: where are we? what next? *Journal of Health and Social Behavior*, **36**(5), 53–79.

Zola, I.K. (1972) Medicine as an institution of social control. *Sociological Review*, **20**(4), 487–504.

# Chapter 8

# SPORT, HEALTH AND STEROIDS: PARADOX, CONTRADICTION OR ETHICAL SELF-FORMATION?

Helen Keane

## Introduction

This chapter examines the relationship between health and sport, focusing on the practices of bodybuilders who use anabolic steroids. Bodybuilding is a marginalised and frequently demonised sporting subculture, very different from more mainstream sports in social position and cultural meaning. Despite its distinctiveness, it is often referred to in general accounts of the paradoxical relationship between sport and health, and it also features prominently in critiques of sport as an institution which reproduces gender inequality. For example, for feminist scholars Gillett and White (1992, p.358), bodybuilding represents 'the male body as the embodiment of physical power'. Following recent ethnographic studies which challenge such pathologising interpretations, I investigate the practices of bodybuilding as a form of embodied ethical performance (Monaghan, 2001a, b). The notion of ethical performance that I use combines Foucault's understandings of ethics (1985) and the recent work of Simon Williams on the concept and experience of health (1998). It enables a refiguring of steroid use as an element in a specific performance of health, rather than a form of drug abuse or risky behaviour that emerges from underlying individual pathology. This understanding of steroid use has the advantage of reflecting more closely the meanings bodybuilders themselves construct around their substance use and its relationship to their identity and embodiment. It suggests that an over-attachment to paradox and contradiction as organising themes in the analysis of health can overlook the specific logic of different bodily projects.

The chapter begins by reviewing the dominant sociological understanding of the sport–health relationship as a paradox, in which the benefits of physical exercise and pleasures of skilful play are overshadowed by the destructive effects of a competitive and aggressive masculine culture. I argue that this perspective is limited by its focus on hegemonic masculinity and its assumption that health is fundamentally an objective physiological state. Simon Williams' (1998) theorisation of health as a contradictory moral performance is promising for a nuanced understanding of sport and health, as it highlights both the cultural and subjective nature of health. It also emphasises that health is not a singular condition or abstract ideal but an experience and identity enacted through concrete activities, such as exercise and sport. However, Williams' notion of health retains a binary structure, in which health as discipline is contrasted with health as transgression (1998, p.441). This may illuminate some of the dilemmas produced by the demand and desire to be healthy, but it cannot capture the hybrid nature of a practice like bodybuilding.

Combining William's insight about health as performance with Foucault's model of ethics as a process of self-formation provides a more flexible way of examining the meaning of bodybuilding practice (and other sporting activity). The final part of the chapter draws on interviews with male steroid-using bodybuilders carried out in Sydney, Australia, to present an account of bodybuilding as a form of ethical performance. Three themes emerged as key elements in the bodybuilders' self-construction as ethical subjects – physical growth and personal transformation; dedication and the use of time; and health as distinction. While the bodybuilders interviewed did not emphasise masculinity when reflecting on the meaning of and motivation for their bodily practices, their appreciation of muscular embodiment as a manifestation of dedication and willpower places high value on the capacity of the male body to change and grow.

## Sport and health as paradox

Paradox has become a structuring motif in the social scientific literature on sport and its relationship to health (Messner, 2005). On one hand, the status of sport as an activity which promotes wellbeing is both scientifically endorsed and symbolically reinforced (Fox, 1999). The sportive body represents health as strength, stamina, agility and competence. In a visual culture where health is constructed as the attainment of an ideal body type, the toned and muscular body of the elite athlete is an object of desire and aspiration (Parker, 1996; Miller, 1998). But sport also retains its everyday pedagogic functions. Sporting activity is seen as particularly beneficial for children and youth, promoting virtues such as fitness, discipline, sociability and teamwork; and protecting against the ills of obesity, depression, crime and drug use (Ferron et al., 1999; Ewing et al., 2002). Indeed, the association between sport and good health has been described as an ideology with 'near universal acceptance across a range of societies' (Waddington, 2000, p.408).

On the other hand, playing sport also produces injury and pain, and among high-level athletes intense training and the pressures of competition frequently have detrimental effects on wellbeing (Sabo, 1995; White et al., 1995). The damaged body of the elite athlete – being carried from the field, collapsing during a race, undergoing repeated 'reconstruction' – vividly represents the costs of commitment to sporting excellence. Moreover, for some children, especially boys, sport is an experience dominated by anxiety and humiliation as it marks their bodies as inadequate. Teasing is an under-acknowledged but widely reported aspect of school sport (Markula & Pringle, 2006; Ziviani et al., 2006).

As feminist research has emphasised, sport is a prime site for the construction and reproduction of masculinity, male power and beliefs about the 'natural' attributes of the male body (Birrell, 1988; Messner, 1992; Parker, 1996; Dworkin & Messner, 2000). Thus the benefits and costs of sport are intensified when they are considered specifically in relation to masculinity and the lives of boys and men. Sports such as rugby and cricket were introduced in British public schools in the nineteenth century in order to produce the civilised manliness necessary to lead the empire (Crossett, 1990; Gruneau, 1993). The idea that sport, especially contact team sport, 'makes men' out of boys is still prevalent, with the notion of manhood doing double service as both a natural attribute of male bodies and a desirable state achieved only through dedicated work on the self (Hargreaves, 2000).

While less explicitly concerned with ideals of manhood, contemporary community and government programmes also harness sport in order to improve male conduct. For example, the UK government has used sport in health promotion campaigns as a way of overcoming men's supposed indifference to messages about nutrition and preventive care (Robertson, 2003). In the US, sports programmes have been seen as a way of reducing crime and violence among underprivileged inner-city youth (Coakley, 2002). In this kind of programme, sport is assumed to have a universal appeal and relevance to boys and men, while at the same time being a remedy or outlet for undesirable masculine traits such as aggression, recklessness and lack of care for the self.

In contrast to the view of sport as a route to healthy manhood, the critical sociology of sport and gender has understood the close association between sport and masculinity as detrimental to individual and societal wellbeing. As McKay and colleagues (2000, p.6) have observed, this field has tended to focus on the negative outcomes of the 'male sports experience'. It has highlighted the association of sport with physical trauma, drug and alcohol misuse and the treatment of the body as a machine or tool (Connell, 1990; Sabo, 1995; Messner et al., 2000; Messner, 2002). It sees sport as an institution which maintains a gender regime in which risk-taking and stoicism are essential attributes of masculinity. This ideal of male invulnerability is linked to men's morbidity, lower use of health services and lower life expectancy (Luck et al., 2000).

Beyond the effects of sport on individual men, critical sports studies have highlighted the homophobic, misogynist and racist culture of men's sport (Messner, 2002). Scholars informed by feminism have argued convincingly that male violence both on and off the field is a central and legitimated feature of sport, rather than the unfortunate misbehaviour of a minority of players (Messner et al., 2000). Messner (2002) describes a 'triad of men's violence' that is sustained by the hierarchical homosociality of athletic peer groups: violence against women, violence against other men and violence against the self.

Much of the analysis in critical and feminist accounts of men and sport, especially in relation to violence, is underpinned by the concept of hegemonic masculinity. Developed by R.W. Connell in the 1980s, hegemonic masculinity was quickly taken up and widely applied in masculinity studies (Hearn, 2004, p.56). Hegemonic masculinity refers to a dominant and culturally exalted form of masculinity, 'the currently most honored way of being a man' (Connell & Messerschmidt, 2005, p.832). Hegemonic masculinity is proposed to maintain and legitimate an unequal gender order by subordinating women (and other devalued masculinities). Sport is viewed as a key medium for the reproduction of hegemonic masculinity because of its emphasis on bodily force and physical skill, and its role in the socialisation of boys (Connell, 1983; Miller, 1998; Dworkin & Wachs, 2000).

Hegemonic masculinity has undoubtedly been a productive concept for the study of gender relations in sport. It explains the popularity and cultural endorsement of confrontational contact sports, the acceptance of pain and injury, and the ritualised sexism and homophobia of sporting milieus (Connell & Messerschmidt, 2005). But it has also become a limiting framework. Its pervasiveness has led to the repeated presentation of sport as a static and uniform arena of gender hierarchy. While Connell has stressed the mobility and historicity of hegemonic gender forms, and the importance of recognising diverse masculinities, the use of hegemonic masculinity in sports studies has not reflected this complexity. Rather than a configuration of social practice, hegemonic masculinity has often been deployed as a fixed and abstract ideal type. For example, in a study of adolescent boys' views of masculinity in relation to sport, Laberge and Albert (2000, p.200) describe the boys' understandings of masculinity as approximating 'the hegemonic form'.

The conceptual dominance of hegemonic masculinity has produced a relatively narrow vision of masculinity in sports studies. When different performances of masculinity are considered, they are often understood as alternative forms, while hegemonic masculinity retains its conceptual centrality. In addition, claims about sport in general have been based on evidence from high-profile team sports such as football, rugby and basketball where the privileging of a conventional masculinity based on aggression, toughness and physical power can be readily demonstrated. The heterogeneous ways that sports such as cycling, golf, handball, windsurfing and ice skating produce masculinity and male embodiment have received attention, but insights from these studies are not often incorporated in broader accounts of gender and sport (Wheaton, 2000; Broch, 2003; Butryn & Masucci, 2003; Kestnbaum, 2003; Hundley, 2004).

Accounts of the sports–health paradox thus rest on circumscribed models of masculinity and particular types of sport. They also tend to presume that health costs and health benefits are objectively identifiable entities that can be aggregated and compared. Criticism of the unreflexive celebration of sport as healthy is well developed in sports studies literature, but health is often taken for granted as a universal category. For example, Ivan Waddington (2000) makes a useful distinction between the benefits of 'non-competitive rhythmic exercise' and the more mixed effects of competitive sport on wellbeing. He also criticises the ideology of victim-blaming 'healthism' which often accompanies statements extolling the benefits of sport (Waddington, 2000, pp.409, 419). However, his (admittedly brief) review does not include a discussion of the notion of health itself. Physiological measures dominate his list of the health benefits of exercise: cardiovascular function, control of obesity, decreased blood pressure and improved glucose tolerance in diabetes (2000, pp.411–12). The experience and varied meanings of health for embodied subjects, and the connection between an effect like 'decreased blood pressure' or a condition like diabetes and a sense of oneself as healthy remains unexplored.

## From paradox to moral and ethical performance

Unsurprisingly, the sociology of health has been more attentive than sports studies to the significance of health as a regulatory cultural ideal and a subjective experience (Crawford, 1984, 2006; Crossley, 2003). Simon

Williams has advocated a notion of health as moral performance, in which health is not a thing one has or is, but a 'reiterative set of ritualized practices' through which one constructs a viable identity. In this model, the performance of health does not express an underlying physiological status or condition, it constructs the very experience and identity of health. The performance is moral, in Williams' (1998) terms, because in the contemporary West, health is 'a prime site from which claims to social membership are demonstrated' (p.450). In particular, health involves the ritualistic resolution of the contradictory imperatives of discipline and pleasure produced by consumer capitalist society. Reflecting this broader cultural contradiction, health is understood as both bodily control and corporeal transgression. On one hand, healthy citizens control and discipline their bodies in conformity with the latest expert advice. In this mode, health is about work and denial, and its slogan is 'no pain, no gain'. On the other hand, health is also promoted as 'a consuming passion and pleasurable release' where 'a little bit of what you fancy does you good'. In this mode health is about enjoyment and flourishing rather than willpower and restraint (Williams, 1998, pp.440–43).

While Williams (1998) states that the imperatives of control and release are 'inextricably intertwined', his account of their operation suggests an oppositional dichotomy in which understandings of health 'oscillate precariously' between the two extremes of discipline and pleasure. Thus health is viewed primarily as a site of contradiction and dilemma. This binarised model emerges in part from Williams' commitment to an ontology of the body as primordially transgressive and recalcitrant, its unruly appetites and desires resistant to rational control (1998, p.438). But lived experiences of health and body management are more hybrid and heterogeneous than the contrasting categories of discipline/pain and transgression/pleasure suggest. And while contradiction is *one* of the experiences of modern health, individuals do not necessarily experience different modes of embodiment as contradictory. In the corporeal practices of bodybuilding it is difficult to separate discipline from transgression. Intense daily weight training, often targeting a specific muscle, demands discipline and the endurance of pain but it also represents transgressive corporeal excess and produces the pleasures of 'the pump' which occurs when blood fills an overtaxed muscle. Moreover, bodybuilders often describe the rigours of training as an escape from the more complex requirements of work and relationships, the pain and intensity enhancing rather than hindering the experience of release.

A Foucauldian understanding of ethics provides one way of thinking outside the binaries of paradox and contradiction in relation to bodily practices. In the second volume of his history of sexuality, *The Use of Pleasure*, Foucault (1985) draws on ancient Greek texts to reconstruct a mode of ethics which focuses on self-formation rather than adherence to an explicit moral code. From this perspective the goal of an ethical life is to form oneself into an ethical subject, through the development of the correct attitude to oneself and one's pleasures. In the example of the Greeks, Foucault saw the possibility of an ethic without the assumption of a prior human subject, without a universal moral code and free from the normalisation such a code implies.

Foucault's concepts of creative self-constitution and ethical practice enable an account of health that recognises its moral significance but which is not based on an idealised vision of 'perfect' health nor attached to a normative model of the human body and its functioning. For example, approaching health in terms of ethical self-formation does not assume that longevity is the universal measure of wellbeing, nor that 'the natural body' has a privileged relationship to health. Neither does it presume a pre-existing ontology of discipline versus corporeal excess. It enables recognition of the reflective and ethical content of a practice such as steroid-assisted bodybuilding that may appear to outsiders to be nothing but reckless self-harm. Exploring the varied way that the requirements of ethical self-formation are addressed by different embodied practices moves us beyond the designation of people's relations to their bodies as simply healthy/ unhealthy. Rather we can analyse performances of health in terms of their own objects, relations and goals. This is not necessarily to endorse such practices as health enhancing in an objective sense, but to recognise their internal logic and ethical content.

## Bodybuilding as ethical practice and performance

As I have already noted, the most influential literature on masculinity and sport has been based on studies of sports such as football and basketball. These sports are characterised by their status as arenas of homosociality and hypercompetitive masculine performance, their exalted place in the 'sports industrial complex' and their conferring of social privilege. In contrast, bodybuilding is a marginal sport, one that has been insightfully analysed as a 'demonised subculture' (Monaghan, 2001a, b). However, in common with mainstream team sports, it has been understood by critical and feminist scholars as a vehicle of hegemonic masculinity. The exaggerated muscularity of the bodybuilder has been seen as a literalised celebration of masculine power, in which muscles signify patriarchy (Gillett &

White, 1992). In addition, Gillett and White (1992) argue that the body-builder is caught in a paradoxical relationship to power, in which he becomes dependent on the pursuit of an idealised image which is never achieved. Alan Klein's widely cited ethnographic study presents an equally pathologised vision of bodybuilders as 'little big men' whose obsession with size emerges from masculine insecurity:

> Seeking to be large is, for the bodybuilder, a defence against the thing he fears most of all, his smallness. This has clear implications not only for his fragile ego structure but also for his gender identity structure, which is also shaky. (Klein, 1995, p.115)

This compensatory account of bodybuilding has been critiqued by Lee Monaghan (2001b) whose recent work systematically explores the meaning of bodybuilding from the bodybuilder's perspective. Monaghan argues convincingly that bodybuilders are, like many citizens of late modernity, involved in ongoing projects of embodied identity production which draw on technological (including biochemical) resources. Fundamental to the bodybuilding project and the subcultural participation that it entails is the cultivation of a new way of looking at the muscular body involving a unique aesthetic code. In the culture of bodybuilding, the muscular body is not an undifferentiated object which signifies patriarchal masculinity, but a range of embodied styles reflecting varied projects of self-development. Therefore, the bodybuilder's appreciation of the muscular body is not an expression of pathology, but rather an acquired cultural taste (Monaghan, 1999a). In relation to steroid use, without denying potential harm, Monaghan highlights the value placed by bodybuilders on 'correct' use based on technical competence and careful planning of 'cycles' (Monaghan, 2001a, b).

In what follows, my aim is to extend Monaghan's analysis by considering steroid-assisted bodybuilding as a form of ethical performance which produces a specific form of healthy embodiment. I draw on 15 interviews I carried out with male steroid-using bodybuilders in Sydney, Australia, in 2001. The interviews, which were part of a larger study of steroid use and the meaning and experience of health, were between 1.5 and 2 hours long and were fully transcribed. The men ranged in age from 21 to 45. All except one, who described himself as Greek, were Anglo-Australians. They had various occupations including teaching, community and social work, trades, and hospitality. The majority were non-competitive bodybuilders, although one had competed in the past, one was currently competing, and one was aiming to compete in the future. The approach taken to the interviews was broadly phenomenological, that is, they aimed to elucidate the meaning of building a muscular body through reflective description of the patient's own experiences and daily life. However, the narratives were not taken at face value; the themes which were identified from the transcripts were analysed using the framework of Foucauldian ethics and health as moral performance outlined earlier.

The interview narratives constituted bodybuilding as a project of self-construction, built around a complex regime of bodily micromanagement focused on exercise, rest, regulated eating and nutritional and pharmacological supplementation. Participants have different levels of attachment to bodybuilding, and the intensity of their involvement tends to vary over time. Nevertheless, for serious participants, bodybuilding involves the construction and ongoing performance of an embodied identity which emphasises the connection between internal qualities and the external appearance of the body. In the narratives of bodybuilders, becoming an ethical subject with a correct relationship to one's body involves the replacement of ignorance and immaturity with specialised knowledge and discipline. Adherence to the bodybuilding regime produces a performative identity based not only on muscular embodiment but on a critical and reflective relationship with one's body and one's self.

## Physical growth and personal transformation in bodybuilding

In terms of Foucauldian ethics, the most obvious substance of the body-builder's project is his muscles, their mass, shape, symmetry and definition. As Monaghan has demonstrated, bodybuilders differentiate between types of muscular body and evaluate them according to aesthetic appeal. The attainment of sheer size is rejected as a proper goal for those wishing to achieve a 'quality' physique (Monaghan, 1999a, p.273). An experienced bodybuilder linked his preferred style with a feminine sensibility:

**Darren**: I'm into aesthetically pleasing. I like . . . the good nice tapered shape and all that kind of stuff. I'm not really into density or thickness, but that's just a personal thing. Um, I perhaps look at it, for want of better expression, from a female point of view, or what I perceive as a female point of view. 'Wow, that's a really symmetrically looking great body', not a big nugget which has got the most mass.

Despite Darren's critique, increasing mass is a crucial element of body-building and anabolic steroids are utilised for their ability to promote muscle accumulation through protein synthesis. Describing the motivations for their training and steroid use, the bodybuilders emphasised the *process* of physical growth over the attainment of a goal size or weight. The satisfaction of observing one's body developing was highlighted:

**Jake**: It's like watching a baby grow. It's just the way it all comes along, like, watching yourself grow and taking shape.

Jake's metaphor of infant development constructs the process as the unfolding of an inherent and natural potential within the individual, while also emphasising the consistent and extended effort required to produce a healthy child (or impressive body). His training partner and mentor who was interviewed at the same time, added:

**Rob**: If you're a sprinter, you have achieved such and such a time . . . But when you wake up in the morning, and you see yourself in the mirror you don't say 'Oh, look, there's that wonderful sprinter'. But when you are a bodybuilder, you see those results, you wake up in the morning and – 'God, you've got a great body' – the results are there, they're concrete and obvious, it's visual.

However, Rob stressed that the bodybuilder's pleasure in the spectacle of his body was not simple narcissism. Like most of the participants, he spoke passionately about the development of self-discipline through the demands of bodybuilding:

**Rob**: You gain discipline through the actual experience. Yes, the more knowledge you have about it, the more disciplined you become because you know what it entails to gain success, you need to be disciplined. You need to follow things through to the end. If you don't do that, well then you're not going to achieve. And you know that. So, as a result of that . . . well, you know that if you don't eat, you won't grow. You know that if you don't take your anabolic steroids at a certain time, you won't grow.

Thus hypermuscularity is valued as a visual reflection of discipline and evidence of the correct application of training techniques. Muscle becomes an ethical substance in this context because it is a materialisation of the mastery of the self that develops from adherence to a rigorous regime. Rather than a generalised symbol of hegemonic masculinity, the built body is decoded by bodybuilders as a signifier of expertise and ethical growth.

The particular performance of health enacted by and recognised by body-builders privileges self-willed corporeal transformation, a process that is experienced as both pleasurable and demanding. Developing a spectacular physique has significance as an exercise of will because, as one respondent remarked, 'the body doesn't like changing, it doesn't matter what you put into it, it doesn't like changing' [Spencer].

While none of the participants identified the capacity for self-willed change as a unique characteristic of men or the male body, the rendering of muscle as an ethical substance is clearly productive of a hierarchical gender difference. As Helen Gremillion (2002) has argued, the female body is regarded in contemporary popular and medical discourse as an obstacle to fitness: men are encouraged to *stay fit*, while women are encouraged to *get fit*. A similar valorisation of the male body and its ability to harden and grow in response to training is found in bodybuilding discourse. But at the same time the pharmacology of bodybuilding can produce an awareness of the male body as hormonal and labile, which highlights sexual similarity rather than sexual difference. Indeed, a number of participants compared their use of steroids with the use of hormonal contraceptives and medications by women.

Given the link made between physical growth and ethical status, the idea that steroid use could substitute for hard work in the gym was vehemently dismissed. While recognising that drug use contributed to the results they achieved, several interviewees stressed that without proper training and nutrition, steroids had little effect. Rejection of the mainstream view of steroid use as cheating enabled bodybuilders to incorporate pharmacological enhancement into their ethical projects of disciplined self-production. A personal trainer and martial arts practitioner explained his steroid use as pragmatic (assisting his training and recovery from injury) but also as an integral part of his relationship to himself as a project: 'I'm doing it [using steroids] for myself; I'm trying to test myself. What is my true potential? Where does my ultimate limit lie?' [Brett]. Rather than artificial enhancement, Brett saw steroids as enabling him to transcend the arbitrary limits of embodiment and contingent obstacles such as the need to earn a living, in order to become the best possible version of himself.

## Dedication and the use of time

The significance of the ideal of dedication in bodybuilding has been well documented (Fussell, 1991; Klein, 1993; Monaghan, 2001a, b). Dedication entails sacrificing the flexibility and pleasures of 'normal life' for a gruelling routine and commitment to goals that are viewed as bizarre by outsiders. Diet and the avoidance of alcohol were key elements of dedication which arose in the interviews. The diet described by Spencer, a competitive bodybuilder who had been in the sport for 20 years, demonstrates a form of consumption that constitutes food as fuel and eschews the social world of meals:

**Before morning training**: black coffee.

**After training**: 250 g chicken breast, sweet corn, sweet potato, cauliflower, Brussels sprouts

**Two hours later**: 100 g rolled oats cooked in water, 12 egg whites

**Three hours later**: canned tuna, 1.5 cups rice

**After evening training**: salad, turkey breast

**Before bed**: canned tuna

While the diets outlined by other bodybuilders were not as precise or restricted, weighing food and eating 5 or 6 times a day was common, and nearly all said they aimed to eat a large amount of protein and limit fat and carbohydrates. Neil, a bodybuilder in his mid 30s who had used steroids for five years, described training as 'all about numbers – how many reps, how many calories, how many mils . . . everything is broken down into three things besides sleep' [Neil]. Because 'three things besides sleep' (training, nutrition and steroid cycles) become 'everything', the ethical work of bodybuilding concerns what is sacrificed as well as what is endured. Social life is restricted by diet and training schedules, recreation is limited and relationships, finances and job opportunities often suffer. Will, who had a full-time job in health services and was also in the army reserve, described his life in training as 'a sort of solitary exile'. But he followed his account of the pleasures he had to forgo with an assessment of these pleasures as ultimately less gratifying than the benefits of 'staying home and not drinking, getting adequate sleep, not wasting money on alcohol'. Thus, the meaning of sacrifice could be inverted by constituting everyday pastimes and desires as deficient in genuine value or meaning.

While the ideal of dedication requires devoting substantial time to bodybuilding, the efficient use of this time emerged from the interviews as a key characteristic of the bodybuilding ethos. Aidan said he went to the gym every day but stressed that 'I'm not the kind of person who spends hours there . . . you can get a decent exercise, a workout, over and done with within half an hour or 45 minutes . . . just get in there, do it, and then leave' [Aidan]. Rob also mentioned the importance of an intense workout of 1.5 hours maximum 'because this is not a marathon' [Rob]. The efficiency, intensity and focus of bodybuilding was contrasted with the leisurely 'time-wasting and chatting' approach of other fitness activities such as aerobics, stationery bikes and treadmills. In bodybuilding narratives 'efficiency' and 'waste' were not objective evaluations of time use, but categories of meaning which contrasted the focus necessary to achieve specific and concrete goals with a vague desire to 'get fit'. For example, Colin mentioned watching television while exercising, a popular pastime in commercial gyms, as a prime example of poor time use. While combining another activity with exercise could be interpreted as efficient multitasking, from his perspective it demonstrated a lack of dedication to the serious work of training.

The goal of efficiency had particular salience because efficiency depends on the specialised knowledge of physiology and nutrition necessary to achieve maximum growth in minimum time. Wasting time therefore represented the antithesis of bodybuilding ethics because it symbolised a lack of respect for oneself and one's body. In contrast, steroid use could acquire positive ethical value because it enhanced efficiency. For Will, steroid use was all about time management:

**HK**: So the ideal that you're aiming for is what you had before, with the steroids. Do you think you could achieve that ideal without them?

**Will**: I could, if I stopped working and allowed myself to train and do an hour and a half or an hour 5 or 6 days a week, and not work so much. You just need so much time. You need time to rest because you're on the go all the time . . . So if I wasn't working and had lots more time, then I could achieve it. It takes a lot longer training as well. In 3 months, with the aid of a course of steroids, I can do what would take me 6 or 9 months or probably even longer without them – and I just don't have that time. That's a year of concentrated training.

The beneficial effects of anabolic steroids on time management were also described with enthusiasm by Colin. He linked steroids not just to improved performance at the gym, but a global sense of efficiency and achievement:

**Colin:** You can just get a lot more done. You probably are thinking faster; you're a lot more confident. If you want to say something, you just say it. It seems like everyone's sort of there and you're up here . . . When you're a quiet person and you're on a cycle, you're sort of loud, better at doing things. Like you can train for 2 hours and then come home and you can mow the lawn after that, if you want, and then after that you can go for a walk for an hour.

Time was experienced by the bodybuilders as a resource in short supply whose limited availability impeded their progress. It was also constructed as a resource that should be actively managed as part of a goal-oriented life. Therefore anabolic steroids were seen as a legitimate and rational training aid rather than a means of artificial enhancement.

## Health as distinction

Although anabolic steroid use was recognised as a potentially risky practice, the bodybuilders saw the built body as exemplifying a specific but highly desirable form of health. The respondents constructed themselves as drug-using but ethical subjects by contrasting their own health and body management with two groups characterised by their lack of discipline and insight: irresponsible bodybuilders and the 'general population'.

Ethnopharmacological expertise, a detailed subcultural understanding of the properties of different steroids, dosages, administration routes and cycling theory (how to combine periods of steroid use and non-use to maximise gains) was central to the distinction between health-conscious bodybuilding and irresponsible health-damaging bodybuilding (Monaghan, 1999b). Martin, a personal trainer and aspiring actor, contrasted his carefully researched steroid cycles with the chaotic and excessive consumption of 'guys in the gym who want to be the biggest':

**Martin:** [I get my knowledge] from books and the Internet . . . I mean, guys in the gym will just say 'Look, man, I'm taking 2 grams of testosterone and threw 4 anabol down my system' and that's a potent oral drug that goes passing through the liver and this is what's giving guys the side effects. It's this drug; what it can do in size and strength is unbelievable. So these guys take 4 or 5 a day and they kill themselves.

The interviewees argued that side effects, including 'roid rage', could be avoided through the controlled but effective drug use made possible by the intelligent application of ethnopharmacological knowledge. From this perspective, the disciplined subjectivity produced by a dedication to body-building itself acts as a protection against the harmful effects of steroids.

**HK**: So do you think it's true that steroids make you aggressive, the idea of 'roid rage'? Is that valid?

**Martin**: Only if it's within you before you started the cycle. If you're on alcohol and you take steroids, you're in big trouble. You're going to kill someone. But if you're a calm person and you're on the level, and if you're into sports and progress, I think you'll be right. I think you'll love being on them and you'll feel incredible.

While the excesses of some bodybuilders were criticised, the ignorance, laziness and lack of self-care demonstrated by 'the average person' were also disparaged.

**Will**: Most people don't know . . . know hardly anything about nutrition, about what they put in their mouth every day, about the detrimental effects that certain lifestyles and habits are doing to them – like smoking or drinking Coke every day in terms of dental hygiene and stuff. Even just sitting on your bum in an office job all day and not exercising, or not so much detrimental to your health, it's just you feel so much better if you do get out and perform some sort of exercise and training.

**Aidan**: Most people are oblivious. I think in general most people have no idea. Most people, girls don't eat properly. And you can tell, every girl I've ever met has been constipated and it takes like a week or two before you teach them how to eat properly . . . Most guys drink too much and you watch, they get to about 30 and then they just, they go from these young guys that look good to just dying. No I don't think people are healthy at all.

Mainstream health experts were blamed for spreading misinformation about diet and exercise (and steroids) which was blindly accepted by the public. Dedicated to high protein diets, the bodybuilders criticised 'dieticians who say we shouldn't be eating meat and make us want to turn ourselves into sheep' [Tim] and the promotion of carbohydrates as healthy food [Rob]. Health centres were derided for promoting gimmicks such as pump classes while failing to teach proper weight-training technique. Of aerobics instructors, Colin said 'they just don't look healthy, they've got no muscle tone and they're very flat. They might be able to jump around and that for 45 minutes but I can do that anyway'.

By highlighting the commodified and consumerist nature of mainstream fitness culture, the bodybuilders enhanced their moral performance as adherents to a purer and deeper pursuit of wellbeing. Immersion in a subculture commonly involves distancing oneself from the uninitiated masses. But in the case of bodybuilding, the performance of a particular subcultural ethics also involves refiguring health as *distinction*. That is, the bodily practices and corporeal aesthetics of bodybuilding gain value for participants because they are not normal or standard, but exclusive. They transform health into an optimum physicality attainable only through extreme dedication and discipline, not something that can be incorporated into ordinary, everyday life.

Bodybuilders recognise that their desired style of embodiment is highly specialised, and they value this specialisation even though it may diminish rather than enhance some aspects of everyday functioning. Tim explained that although he had put on 20 kg of muscle and was much healthier and stronger since committing to bodybuilding, he was less able to do ordinary heavy lifting.

**Tim**: Your body learns to focus on training only a particular muscle over a particular time and loses the idea of how to use them all together. So, picking up that television, you've got to grab hold of it, hug it, heave . . . right? Whereas what will happen to me is I'll get a vice-like grip on it with my hands but it will actually be quite difficult for me to manoeuvre.

In its celebration of specialisation and exclusivity, the ethics of bodybuilding is a challenge to dominant discourses of health and wellbeing which promote health as the outcome of a 'balanced lifestyle', a state attainable by everyone through relatively undemanding practices of moderation. As Emily Martin (1998) has argued, contemporary western cultures place a high value on flexibility and adaptability: a body and subjectivity which is fluid and open to change has become the epitome of health and fitness. But counter-discourses and subcultures of health, such as bodybuilding, which value a different mode of 'vibrant physicality' exist and flourish (Monaghan, 2001b). For participants in these subcultures the global ideal of fitness and productivity is traded for a corporeal ethic of dedication, distinction and transformation.

## Conclusion

Assessments of the relationship between health and sport have commonly balanced the benefits of sport such as cardiovascular fitness and weight control against costs such as injury and stress. Because sport has both positive and negative effects on wellbeing, the relationship is viewed as paradoxical. But if health is recognised as a subjective experience and culturally loaded performance of identity rather than an objective and primarily physiological state, the interplay between sport and health becomes more complex and less open to generalisation. This chapter has argued that the Foucauldian notion of ethics as self-formation is a productive tool for the analysis of sporting practices and their connection with the moral performance of health. In the case of male bodybuilders who use anabolic steroids, the ethical perspective undermines the interpretation of their corporeal manipulation as reckless and pathological self-harm which emerges from gender insecurity. Instead it constitutes bodybuilding as a project of self-formation in which controlled drug use is valued as a sign of expertise, discipline and dedication. This is not to deny that steroid use can be harmful, nor that a dedication to bodybuilding and its narrow definition of success can produce a precarious sense of self. However, for participants, accepting these risks is not paradoxical, because the risks are integral to the distinctive and demanding model of health they aim to perform as dedicated bodybuilders.

## References

Birrell, S.J. (1988) Discourses on the gender/sport relationship: from women in sport to gender relations. *Exercise and Sport Science Reviews*, **16**(1), 459–502.

Broch, H.B. (2003) Embodied play and gender identities in competitive handball for children in Norway. In: *Sport, Dance and Embodied Identities* (eds N. Dyck & E.P. Archetti), pp.75–93. Oxford; New York: Berg.

Butryn, T. & Masucci, M. (2003) It's not about the book: a cyborg counternarrative of Lance Armstrong. *Journal of Sport and Social Issues*, **27**(2), 124–144.

Coakley, J. (2002) Using sports to control deviance and violence among youths: let's be critical and cautious. In: *Paradoxes of Youth and Sport* (eds M. Gatz, M.A. Messner & S.J. Ball-Rokeach), pp.13–30. Albany, NY: State University of New York Press.

Connell, R.W. (1983) *Which Way is Up? Essays on Sex, Class, and Culture.* Sydney: Allen & Unwin.

Connell, R.W. (1990) An iron man: the body and some contradictions of hegemonic masculinity. In: *Sport, Men and the Gender Order* (eds M. Messner & D. Sabo), pp.83–96. Champaign, IL: Human Kinetics.

Connell, R.W. & Messerschmidt, J.W. (2005) Hegemonic masculinity: rethinking the concept. *Gender and Society*, **19**(6), 829–859.

Crawford, R. (1984) A cultural account of 'health': control, release and the social body. In: *Issues in the Political Economy of Health Care* (ed. J. McKinlay), pp.60–103. London: Tavistock.

Crawford, R. (2006) Health as a meaningful social practice. *Health*, **10**(4), 401–420.

Crossett, T. (1990) Masculinity, sexuality and the development of early modern sport. In: *Sport, Men and the Gender Order* (eds M.A. Messner & D. Sabo), pp.45–54. Champaign, IL: Human Kinetics.

Crossley, M.L. (2003) 'Would you consider yourself a healthy person?': using focus groups to explore health as a moral phenomenon. *Journal of Health Psychology*, **8**(5), 501–514.

Dworkin, S.L. & Messner, M.A. (2000) Just do . . . what? Sports, bodies and gender. In: *Revisioning Gender* (eds J. Lorber, B. Hess & M.M. Ferree), pp.341–364. Walnut Creek, CA: AltaMira Press.

Dworkin, S.L. & Wachs, F.L. (2000) The morality/manhood paradox: masculinity, sport, and the media. In: *Masculinities, Gender Relations, and Sport* (eds J. McKay, M.A. Messner & D. Sabo), pp.47–66. Thousand Oaks, CA: Sage Publications.

Ewing, M.E., Gano-Overway, L.A., Branta, C.F. & Vern, D.S. (2002) The role of sports in youth development. In: *Paradoxes of Youth and Sport* (eds M. Gatz, M.A. Messner & S.J. Ball-Rokeach), pp. 31–48. Albany, NY: State University of New York Press.

Ferron, C., Narring, F., Cauderay, M. & Michaud, P-A. (1999) Sport activity in adolescence: associations with health perceptions and experimental behaviours. *Health Education Research*, **14**(2): 225–233.

Foucault, M. (1985) *The Use of Pleasure*. New York: Pantheon Books.

Fox, K.R. (1999) The influence of physical activity on mental well-being. *Public Health Nutrition*, **2**(3a), 411–418.

Fussell, S. (1991) *Muscle: Confessions of an Unlikely Bodybuilder*. New York: Poseidon Press.

Gillett, J. & White, P.G. (1992) Male bodybuilding and the reassertion of hegemonic masculinity: a critical feminist perspective. *Play and Culture*, **5**(4), 358–369.

Gremillion, H. (2002) In fitness and in health: constructing bodies in the treatment of anorexia nervosa. *Signs*, **27**(2), 381–414.

Gruneau, R. (1993) The critique of sport in modernity: theorising power, culture, and the politics of the body. In: *The Sports Process: A Comparative and Developmental Approach* (eds E. Dunning, J. Maguire & R.E. Pearton), pp.85–109. Champaign, IL: Human Kinetics.

Hargreaves, J. (2000) Gender, morality and the national physical education curriculum. In: *Sports, Body and Health* (eds J. Hansen & N.K. Nielsen), pp.133–148. Odense, Denmark: Odense University Press.

Hearn, J. (2004) From hegemonic masculinity to the hegemony of men. *Feminist Theory*, **5**(1), 49–72.

Hundley, H. (2004) Keeping the score: the hegemonic everyday practices in golf. *Communication Reports*, **17**.

Kestnbaum, E. (2003) *Culture on Ice: Figure Skating and Cultural Meaning*. Middletown, CT: Wesleyan University Press.

Klein, A.M. (1993) *Little Big Men: Bodybuilding Subculture and Gender Construction*. Albany, NY: State University of New York Press.

Klein, A.M. (1995) Life's too short to die small: steroid use among male bodybuilders. In: *Men's Health and Illness: Gender, Power and the Body* (eds D. Sabo and D.F. Gordon), pp.105–120. Thousand Oaks, CA: Sage Publications.

Laberge, S. & Albert, M. (2000) Conceptions of masculinity and gender transgressions in sports among adolescent boys: hegemony, contestation, and the social dynamic. In: *Masculinities, Gender Relations, and Sport* (eds J. McKay, M.A. Messner & D. Sabo), pp.195–221. Thousand Oaks, CA: Sage Publications.

Luck, M., Bamford, M. & Williamson, P. (2000) *Men's Health: Perspectives, Diversity, and Paradox*. Oxford; Malden, MA: Blackwell Science.

Markula, P. & Pringle, R. (2006) *Foucault, Sport and Exercise: Power, Knowledge and Transforming the Self*. London; New York: Routledge.

Martin, E. (1998) Flexible bodies: science and new cultures of health in the US. In: *Theorising Medicine, Health and Society* (eds S. Williams, J. Gabe & M. Calnan). London: Sage Publications.

McKay, J., Messner, M.A. & Sabo, D. (2000) Studying sports, men, and masculinities from feminist standpoints. In: *Masculinities, Gender Relations, and Sport* (eds J. McKay, M.A. Messner & D. Sabo), pp.1–12. Thousand Oaks, CA: Sage Publications.

Messner, M.A. (1992) *Power at Play: Sports and the Problem of Masculinity*. Boston, MA: Beacon Press.

Messner, M.A. (2002) *Taking the Field: Women, Men and Sports*. Minneapolis, MN: University of Minnesota Press.

Messner, M.A. (2005) Still a man's world? Studying masculinities and sport. In: *Handbook of Studies on Men and Masculinities* (eds M.S. Kimmel, J. Hearn & R.W. Connell), pp.313–325. Thousand Oaks, CA: Sage Publications.

Messner, M.A., Dunbar, M. & Hunt, D. (2000) The televised sports manhood formula. *Journal of Sport and Social Issues*, **24**(4), 380–394.

Miller, T. (1998) Commodifying the male body, problematizing 'hegemonic masculinity?' *Journal of Sport and Social Issues*, **22**(4), 431–446.

Monaghan, L. (1999a) Creating 'the perfect body': a variable project. *Body and Society*, **5**(2–3), 267–290.

Monaghan, L. (1999b) Challenging medicine? Bodybuilding, drugs and risk. *Sociology of Health and Illness*, **21**(6), 707–734.

Monaghan, L.F. (2001a) *Bodybuilding, Drugs and Risk*. London: Routledge.

Monaghan, L.F. (2001b) Looking good, feeling good: the embodied pleasures of vibrant physicality. *Sociology of Health and Illness*, **23**(3), 330–356.

Parker, A. (1996) Sporting masculinities: gender relations and the body. In: *Understanding Masculinities* (ed. M. Mac an Ghaill). Buckingham, UK: Open University Press.

Robertson, S. (2003) 'If I let a goal in, I'll get beat up': Contradictions in masculinity, sport and health. *Health Education Research*, **18**(6), 706–716.

Sabo, D. (1995) Pigskin, patriarchy and pain. In: *Men's Lives* (eds M.S. Kimmel & M.A. Messner), pp.99–101. Needham Heights, MA: Allyn & Bacon.

Waddington, I. (2000) Sport and health: a sociological perspective. In: *Handbook of Sports Studies* (eds J. Coakley & E. Dunning), pp.408–421. London: Sage Publications.

Wheaton, B. (2000) 'New lads'? Masculinities and the 'new sport' participant. *Men and Masculinities*, **2**(4), 434–456.

White, P.G., Young, K. & McTeer, W.G. (1995) Sport, masculinity, and the injured body. In: *Men's Health and Illness: Gender, Power, and the Body* (eds D. Sabo & D.F. Gordon), pp.158–182. Thousand Oaks, CA: Sage Publications.

Williams, S.J. (1998) Health as moral performance: ritual, transgression and taboo. *Health*, **2**(4), 435–457.

Ziviani, J., McDonald, D., Jenkins, D., Rodger, S., Batch, J. & Cerin, E. (2006) Physical activity of young children. *OTJR: Occupation, Participation and Health*, **26**(1), 4–15.

# Chapter 9

# RACIALISED MASCULINITIES AND THE HEALTH OF IMMIGRANT AND REFUGEE MEN

Bob Pease

## Introduction

In the last 10 years, there has been extensive research on the relationship between masculinity and men's health. However, when health practitioners and policy-makers began to recognise that men's everyday lives were gendered and that their masculine identities had implications for their health, they embraced either biological or sex role theories to explain men's experiences. As I have noted elsewhere (Pease, 1999), sex role theory has replaced the biomedical model in health promotion as the predominant theoretical framework for understanding men's health issues. In response to the limitations of this approach, some critical masculinity scholars have emphasised the importance of locating men's health in the context of class-based, racialised masculinities (see for example Pease, 1999; Connell, 2000; Schofield et al., 2000; Courtenay, 2002; White, 2002; Riska, 2006). Clearly, if men are socially and culturally formed, their health needs will be diverse. Thus in the context of multiple masculinities, some male groups will have specific health needs because they are positioned in different locations in the gendered social divisions of society (Sabo, 2005). However, there have been very few attempts to articulate in detail what this potential stratification in men's experiences might mean for how we understand the relationship between illness and masculinity.

In this chapter, I advocate a gender relations approach to refugee and immigrant men's health (Sabo, 1999, 2005; Schofield et al., 2000; Connell, 2000) that is also informed by critical race theory (Brown, 2003) and intersectional feminism (Mullins & Schulz, 2006). A gender relations approach to health issues emphasises the importance of locating men's health within the context of a diversity of masculinities and unequal gender relations with women. This approach is consistent with what Bentley (2007) calls a 'socially just primary health care', that is able to address the roles that class, race, ethnicity and sexuality play in the health issues facing men. This chapter also builds upon those developments in social science that are concerned with the ways in which men's lives are shaped by the inter-sections of gender, race and class. My aim is to show how masculinity, in interaction with racial and ethnic identification and social class, creates particular health risks for men who are not white. In addressing these links between ethnicity, culture and masculinity in relation to men's health, I will focus on the health needs of refugee and immigrant men.[1]

Understanding the health issues facing refugee and immigrant men requires an analysis of the intersections of both general men's health, and general refugee and migrant health. Most health disparities research addresses gender and race separately. There is insufficient research on men's health which explores the experiences of immigrant and refugee men, and very little of existing research on migrant and refugee health explores gender or masculinity. I will thus explore the limitations of each of these disciplinary areas for understanding the health of refugee and immigrant men, before examining how feminist intersectional analysis, critical masculinity studies and critical race theory can shed new light on the health issues faced by these men.

## The new men's health

In traditional approaches to men's health promotion, individual men are asked to reassess their masculinity and their identity as men and engage in lifestyle changes and preventive healthcare measures. The responsibility for men's health rests with the individual man. If men change their behaviours and attitudes, adopt healthier lifestyles, see their doctors more often and look after their bodies, it is said that they will improve their health (Watson, 2000). These approaches to health promotion portray health as

---

[1] I will not attempt to explore the issue of indigenous men's health as there are very specific issues related to colonialism and dispossession of land that shape the experiences of indigenous groups, and I cannot do justice to the health implications here. Numerous writers have observed significantly greater health problems faced by indigenous men (Pease, 1999; Connell, 2000). Schofield et al. (2000) identify significantly higher rates of premature death among indigenous men with more than 50% of such men not living beyond 50 years of age. I recommend the interested reader to see McCoy's (2004) doctoral thesis where he documents the impact of colonialism on indigenous men's lives through an analysis of petrol sniffing, prison experiences and intergenerational trauma.

something that is largely within the control of the individual male. Men are encouraged to transform their masculinity to lessen the health risks associated with behaviours and to improve the quality of their lives.

If ill-health is a consequence of men's lack of willingness to adopt a healthy lifestyle, then this effectively relieves social institutions of any real responsibility (Wilkinson, 1996). As Doyal (2002, pp.192–3) points out, such changes do not address the 'material and institutional inequalities between men and women that constitute major obstacles to gender equity'. Furthermore, if the source of men's ill-health is located in the gender order, and gender relations need to change, men's interests in maintaining the current arrangements are likely to come to the fore. Men will have to give up privileges associated with their masculinity to improve their lives.

A number of writers have expressed concern about the ways in which men's health issues have been used to position men as the 'new disadvantaged' (Connell, 2000; Whitehead, 2002; Pease, 2006a; Riska, 2006). Whitehead (2002) refers to the portrayal of men's health issues as part of 'the male crisis discourse', which he argues distorts the connections between hegemonic masculinity and men's health. Horrocks (1994, p.1) maintains that 'masculinity in western society is in deep crisis [and that] masculinity is a crisis for men'. In the crisis theory of masculinity, masculinity is portrayed as 'troubled, distracted, counterfeit, constructed, masked, performative, flaccid' (Traister, 2000, p.284). Is masculinity in crisis? Certainly, economic restructuring has challenged working-class men's sense of superiority (McDowell, 2000). In fact, Heartfield (2002) argues that it is the working class, rather than masculinity, that is in crisis. Men have not lost power in relation to women. Rather, both working-class men and women have lost power in relation to the control of their work. Allen (2002) suggests that the idea of masculinity in crisis may itself be a strategy enacted by men to reinforce men's power. As feminists point to the overwhelming evidence of men's disproportionate share of wealth, authority and power, some women find it hard to feel sympathy for the idea of men suffering under male supremacy (Heartfield, 2002).

Even when men's gender privilege is acknowledged, some men's health writers draw attention to the negative psychological effects of this privilege. It is said that men's adherence to hegemonic forms of masculinity have taken a significant health toll on men's lives, leading to a crisis in men's physical and mental health (Coyle & Morgan-Sykes, 1998). Men are thus presented as 'the new victims of advancing, ambitious, driven, sexually-demanding women who are un-attuned and un-attentive to men's needs and who are succeeding often at men's expense' (Coyle & Morgan-Sykes, 1998, p.279).[2]

In Riska's (2006) view, it is the use of the male sex role theoretical framework by men's health theorists that has led to the 'victimization view of men's health'. Connell (2000) argues that this approach to men's health policy lends itself to 'backlash politics' where men's interests are in the forefront of policy development. Such an approach sets itself up against women's health policies by constituting a 'competitive victims discourse'. As I have written about elsewhere (Pease, 1999, 2002), the claim of men's health disadvantage is based on the notion of a homogeneous group of men. Men are not homogeneous but are differentiated by race, ethnicity, class, sexuality and other socio-demographics. Riska (2006) similarly argues that it is only men who are marginalised by race and class who are in crisis, whereas men who are class and race privileged are doing very well in terms of health outcomes. The implication of this is that some groups of white men have excellent standards of healthcare (Schofield et al. 2000).

Schofield (2004, p.20) convincingly points out that men's and women's interests in health are constructed as 'artefacts of an approach based on categorical thinking and quantitative binary comparison'. The basis for the argument that men as a whole are disadvantaged in their health compared to women is highly problematic. The more acute health needs faced by men are more likely to be associated with their class, ethnicity, race or sexuality (Pease, 2002). Riska (2006) has documented, for example, how the focus on men's risk factors for heart disease has neglected the differences in rates of heart disease between men. She notes that this is one of the problems with the social epidemiological approach to sex differences in health outcomes. Gender is operationalised as a dichotomous variable, which does not locate men's health outcomes in the wider social context of the gender order.

Many current policies and programmes addressing men's health issues fail to recognise the social and economic context of men's lives, and the impact of class and race divisions that contribute to their ill-health (Connell, 2000; Pease, 2006a, b; Bentley, 2007). If masculinity is shaped by class and culture, what implications will this have for men's health? Clearly, men who are disadvantaged by class, race and ethnicity are likely to face a wider range of health risks. Because men's

---

[2] See Pease (2006a) for a Foucauldian analysis of government policies in relation to men's health that explores this issue in greater depth.

health and illness varies considerably in relation to class, race, culture, the extent of physical disability and status in the criminal justice system among other factors, men's health promotion should address the issues facing lesser status and marginalised men (Sabo & Gordon, 1995).

We also need to locate men's health within a global context (Wadham, 2001; Courtenay, 2002) and recognise the differential health outcomes for men in different regions of the world. To avoid an essentialist view, we must ensure that the study of men's health emphasises an international perspective. At the same time, we need to be sensitive to the health disparities among men within particular countries. We have to be wary of universalist theories of masculinity that encourage cultural blindness (Seidler, 2006). Seidler (2006) is critical of Connell's notion of hegemonic masculinity because of the implicit premise that it can transcend cultural differences. He emphasises the importance of explaining diversities of masculinities across different cultures (Seidler, 2006). Jones (2006), in a critically important book, has started to fill the gap in our understanding of the lives of ordinary men in the global south, providing an important resource for understanding the relationship between culture and masculinity.

We need to recognise that culture will affect how men develop their masculinities and how they respond to health issues (Luck et al. 2000). Having said that, the dominant norm of masculinity is upheld by a culturally diverse range of men. Barker (2005) demonstrates high levels of commonality in the ways in which diverse cultures define manhood. In my research with immigrant and refugee men, I found that cultural specificity was often used by men to legitimate male privilege and traditional male roles (Pease, 2006b). This has implications for how immigrant and refugee men address their health issues, which I return to later in this chapter.

## The health disparities literature in relation to race and ethnicity

In the health disparities literature, numerous studies compare the health of racial and ethnic minority men and women with that of white men and women (Smedley et al., 2004; Kaytura et al., 2005). In these studies, the health of individuals within particular ethnic groups is compared to the health of whites. Courtenay et al. (2002), for example, explore the extent to which women and men of different ethnic and racial groups manifest different health behaviours and beliefs. Such studies demonstrate that immigrant and refugee men and women have significantly higher risks of receiving poor healthcare. Kennedy and McDonald (2006) document the relationship between unemployment and poorer mental health among immigrants. Asian men in the United Kingdom are shown to have higher rates of heart disease compared to those who are white (Kirby & Kirby, 1999). Also, research shows that such men have higher rates of alcoholism, depression, drug abuse and suicide (Sabo, 2005).

Social epidemiology researches disease and death rates from a perspective that emphasises 'the social distribution and social determinants of states of health' (Lorber & Moore, 2002, p.13). A key debate in the health disparities research is the extent to which disparities in the health outcomes of men and women from non-white ethnic groups can be understood as having genetic versus social causes. Epidemiological studies on the relationship between ethnicity, race and health tend to emphasise the cultural or biological characteristics of men and women within the ethnic or racial group. The majority of research on the links between ethnicity and health takes a 'crude approach to the allocation of individuals within ethnic groups' (Nazroo, 1997, p.9). By focusing on the characteristics of the ethnic group, the causes of ill-health can be found with the culture of the group itself. The concept of health disparities is premised on the measured deviation of marginalised groups' health outcomes from the norms of white people. Such approaches often fail to interrogate the dominant–subordinate relations that shape these unequal outcomes (Weber & Parra-Medina, 2003).

The dominant conception of race in the health sciences literature is thus a biological one (Bhopal, 2007). Weber (2006, p.37) contrasts this biomedical approach to race and health with a 'relational conception of race, class and gender'. She notes that distributional approaches locate difference in men's and women's bodies rather than in gender, class and race relations (Weber, 2006). Mullins and Schulz (2006) also point out how biomedical approaches to health and illness homogenise diversity and difference.

The literature on the social construction of race does not seem to have influenced epidemiological approaches to health and illness. The meaning of racial categories is thus rarely interrogated in epidemiological health inequalities research. Tashiro (2005) raises the concern that the uncritical use of race in health inequalities research can reinforce the view that genetic factors are the major cause of these inequalities. As Mullins and Schulz (2006) comment, much of this literature is based on a typographical approach to health disparities. In this view, genetic differences related to race are regarded as the major factor in explaining differential health outcomes (Mullins & Schulz, 2006). Racial differences in health are thus explained 'in terms of individual biology, genes or behaviour' (Daniels & Schulz, 2006, p.99). Health problems are consequently located in the men's and women's bodies rather than in the context of racial inequalities and institutionalised racism.

One of the ways in which the ideology of race operates is through the belief that it refers to characteristics of individuals who are not white. Hence, whites are constructed as racially invisible and represent the implicit norm against which non-white groups are measured (Tashiro, 2005). So, just as men were historically not seen as gendered in studies of gender and health, white men and women are not seen as racialised in studies of race and health. Rather they are the markers for people of colour (Weber, 2006).

Critical race theorists argue that race is a social category that is invented and reproduced in mundane experiences and customs (Brown, 2003). As a social-constructionist approach to race focuses on how race is constructed and reproduced, this has implications for the links between race and health outcomes. When we theorise race as being socially constructed, it enables us to explore how health outcomes are linked to social, economic and political conditions of men's and women's lives (Daniels & Schulz, 2006). Along with Tashiro (2005), I prefer the term 'racialised populations' to describe these groups. This suggests that race is not an intrinsic quality of individuals but rather something that is imposed on people.

Brown (2003) is one of the few critical race theorists to explore health issues facing immigrant men. She focuses on the mental health difficulties caused by racial stratification. Unlike social epidemiologists who examine only non-white men, she also explores how some mental health problems of white men may be linked with racial stratification. Dysfunctional behaviours and feelings associated with racial prejudice may have psychological health implications for white people. Here the focus is less on ethnicity and culture, and more on the implications of racial stratification for psychological and physical health outcomes of both non-white and white people.

While this chapter is focused on the health issues facing non-white immigrant and refugee men, it is important also to explore the links between whiteness and health. Mullins and Schulz (2006, p.10) draw our attention to the ways in which 'whiteness is constructed in the literatures on racial disparities in health'. It is thus important to recognise how white masculinities are also constructed as racialised identities (Pease, 2004).

## Marginalised masculinities and men's health

The intersection of masculinity with race, class and ethnicity has not been discussed widely in the health disparities literature. Eisler and Herson's

(1999) *Handbook of Gender, Culture and Health* explores various gender and cultural issues associated with health outcomes. However, surprisingly none of the contributors engage with the intersections between culture and gender, let alone between culture and masculinity in relation to health. While there has been some work undertaken on the ways in which class, gender and race relations intersect and are expressed in differential health outcomes for women (Mullins & Schulz, 2006), the challenge is to explore what these intersections might mean for men.

It is clear that men are not equally privileged by patriarchy and that many men are marginalised by race, ethnicity and class (Connell, 1987). Consequently, we need to develop an understanding of the vulnerabilities of marginalised men (Ferguson, 2001). Connell (1995) uses the terms 'marginalised' and 'subordinated' masculinities to describe men who are marginalised by race, class and sexuality. In her view, masculinity is constructed in relation to men's structural location (Connell, 1995). Willis and Porche (2006, p.426) define marginalised men as 'those men who are peripherised on the basis of their identities, associations, experiences and environment'. This includes homeless men, poor men, incarcerated men, unemployed men, mentally ill men, physically disabled men, gay men and immigrant and refugee men. The health needs of such men need to be explored in the context of their specific life circumstances and vulnerabilities. Masculinities marginalised by class, race and ethnicity will be subjected to different influences on men's health.

Stanistreet (2005) is one of the few writers exploring the links between the construction of marginalised men's masculinities and health outcomes. It is the contradiction between hegemonic forms of masculinity and the lived experiences of marginalised men that reproduces men's greater risk-taking to affirm their manhood, which in turn leads to negative health outcomes among such men. Stanistreet (2005) argues that the contradiction between hegemonic masculinity and men's lived experiences reproduces destructive behaviours among marginalised men.

Marginalised men may take greater risks in their efforts to live up to the ideals of hegemonic masculinity. Iacuone (2005) spent six months on building sites as an undisclosed ethnographic researcher exploring the impact of dominant masculine culture on construction workers' attitudes towards occupational health and safety. He observed many cases of risk-taking and dangerous behaviour as the men reinforced their association with idealised conceptions of masculine identity. Men's need to affirm their manhood, it would seem from this study, leads them to take greater risks which in turn, leads to significantly negative health outcomes. Stanistreet (2005, p.16) states that 'the impact of hegemonic masculinity on marginalised men appears to be constructing and sustaining risk taking and self destructive masculinities'. This analysis has implications for how we understand the health of immigrant and refugee men.

How adequate is Connell's (1987) notion of marginalised masculinities for articulating and theorising racialised masculinities? Connell explicitly acknowledges the hierarchies of power whereby non-hegemonic masculinities are marginalised by hegemonic masculinities. By differentiating multiple forms of masculinities, Connell elucidates the relations of power between groups of men. Is this adequate for understanding how masculinities are racialised?

Connell's notion of hegemonic masculinity has been critiqued from various positions over the years (see for example Donaldson, 1993; Jefferson, 1994; Collier, 1998), although none of these critiques have considered its adequacy for understanding the intersections between race and masculinity. Connell herself now acknowledges that her original formulation in *Gender and Power* (1987) that located all masculinities in the context of the global dominance of men over women, failed to do justice to the meaning of multiple masculinities and to men's relations with other men (Connell & Messserschmidt, 2005) but she does not address the issue of concern to us here. She does not, for example, clarify whether she thinks non-white men are racialised outside or inside the relations of power. As such, I argue that race and racism are not adequately conceptualised within Connell's writings in particular or pro-feminist men's writings in general.

In spite of recognising the relevance of race and culture, most pro-feminist writing seems to regard race and culture as peripheral. In discussing the experiences of non-white immigrant and refugee men, they are usually located statistically within structured power relations between men. Race is not considered as being significant in the creation of white masculinities. Rather, race is only an issue that influences the masculinities of non-white men. Thus, I argue that those masculinities that are displayed by marginalised non-white men should not be regarded as a subcategory of the normalised white masculinities.

## Immigrant and refugee men in Australia

While race, ethnicity and geopolitical location are significant influences on health, immigration and refugee status further complicate these intersections. Sayad (1999) talks about what he calls the 'illness of immigration', drawing attention to the ways in which immigrants experience their bodies. Very few studies have examined the health of immigrant and refugee men in Australia (Byrne, 2006). Such research is necessary if we are to understand how men's health problems are influenced by diverse definitions of manhood (Courtenay et al., 2002).

The study of migration has generally ignored the dimensions of gender, assuming that all migrants will have the same experiences of migration. When gender has been examined, it has focused on the experiences of women. In a recent compilation of 31 articles on gender and migration (Willis & Yeoh, 2000), only one article examined the experiences of men (Jones-Correa, 2000). Chambers (1989) noted more than 18 years ago that there had been few attempts to analyse the changing modes of masculinity resulting from migration to Australia, and that we know little about the effects of migration on men's work, leisure and domestic relations. This observation is equally true today.

Immigrant men are more likely than immigrant women to immerse themselves in their own ethnic communities to sustain their status and gendered self image (Jones-Correa, 2000). We can understand this immersion process as a response to racism. Luke (1997), for example, has written about the struggles that Asian men in Australia face when endeavouring to construct masculine identities without the defining characteristics of dominant forms of masculinity. Poynting et al.'s (1998) research with young Lebanese men in Sydney found a highly developed solidarity against 'Aussie' males, that took the form of what Connell (1995) calls 'protest masculinity'. This protest masculinity, which involves exaggerated claims of potency and hypermasculinity, as a result of marginalisation, is similar to the 'cool pose' of African American men discussed by Majors (1989). Similarly, Messner (1997, p.75) discusses how Mexican men in the United States 'displace their class antagonism into the arena of gender relations'. Because they are unable to challenge their class oppressors, Mexican immigrant men display exaggerated expression of masculinity to express power over women within the context of their relative powerlessness. Similar arguments have been advanced about other groups of marginalised and subordinated men. However, in representing aggressive displays of masculinity as a form of resistance against race and class oppression, these studies neglect the impact of their behaviour on women (Messner, 1997).

I am currently undertaking life history research with immigrant and refugee men who have migrated to Australia from four culturally diverse regions of the world: Southern Asia, Southern and East Africa, Latin America and the Middle East. This project is focused on how marginalised and subordinated masculinities are changing in response to refugee experiences, racism and migration. A critical analysis of masculinities in Australia must begin with an analysis of the ways in which marginalised and subordinated masculinities are changing. Immigrant and refugee men are in contradictory positions in relation to dominance and subordination. I am also interested in how a critical examination of immigrant men's masculinities contributes to knowledge about gender-based inequalities in immigrant communities in Australia.

## The social context of immigrant and refugee men's health

Many of the refugee men I interviewed as part of a study on domestic violence in refugee communities (Rees & Pease, 2007) describe stories of economic deprivation, trauma, war, imprisonment and torture. Physical and mental health problems, for example insomnia, anxiety, heightened emotions, worries, reliving and re-experiencing trauma and flashbacks from the past, were directly described. Refugees have necessarily experienced persecution in their country of origin and the number of male participants involved in the study that had experienced trauma and torture in the country of origin was accordingly high. For instance, 47% of men had experienced the murder of a friend or family member, 38% of men had witnessed the murder of a family member or friend, 41% had witnessed torture and 29.4% had experienced torture. Additionally, 41.2% of men had experienced a lack of food or water in the country of origin (Rees & Pease, 2007). This data supports the view that refugee men are necessarily affected by past abuse and hardship in their lives.

Bushra (2000) says that war and disasters have a different impact on women and men because of their different levels of exposure to combat situations. These experiences have a significant impact on their health, including high levels of stress, anxiety and depression. In our study cited above, 17% of men identified feeling depressed 'most of the time'. In a study of Vietnamese refugees in Sydney, Steel et al. (2002) found that such experiences were a major cause of mental illness among refugee men. In relation to some immigrants and refuges, high suicide rates and high levels of mental illness are associated with traumatic experiences and settlement issues (White, 2002).

Similar to the experiences of men of colour in the US, variations in health among immigrant and refugee men in Australia can best be explained by the social and economic context of their lives (Sabo, 2005). Such men are more likely to be economically poor, more likely to live in a polluted environment, and are more likely to work in low paid, dangerous jobs. In this view, we cannot separate ethnicity from the social, economic and historical context of people's lives (Woodward et al., 2001).

Refugee and immigrant men of course are not homogeneous. They are divided by class, religion and sexuality. There is a strong relationship between health and socioeconomic status within particular ethnic groups. Nazroo (1997) argues that socioeconomic position is a more important predictor of health outcomes for members of ethnic groups than ethnicity itself. In his view, we should be less concerned with ethnicity in understanding health variations, and should be more focused on socioeconomic status and health.

There is considerable research demonstrating the impact class divisions have on working-class and immigrant men (see for example White, 2002). Higher rates of diseases associated with the material conditions of working-class men's work and associated higher rates of occupational injuries have been well documented. Men from disadvantaged backgrounds will thus be more likely to experience occupational health hazards and will more likely be involved in violence. Research identifies that men and women in the working class have considerably higher morbidity, mortality and disability rates (Syme & Berkman, 1990). Men on low incomes report their health as fair to poor, at a rate twice that of men on higher incomes (Fletcher, 1995). Working-class men and women generally live in more polluted and crowded environments and in inadequate housing which has a negative effect on their health. Kennedy and McDonald's (2006) study found that unemployment is associated with poorer mental health among immigrants.

When the focus is on men's lifestyles, social class differences are likely to be significant. Research demonstrates that working-class men face more financial difficulties and experience more stressful life events, have access to less social support, and experience greater feelings of disempowerment at work (Kirby & Kirby, 1999). We also know that such men have higher rates of alcohol consumption, drug-taking and smoking, and that they exercise less and have poorer diets. While exercise and nutritional food are seen as being under individual control, disadvantaged men may lack the time to exercise and the money for healthier food (Lorber & Moore, 2002).

Upon arrival, refugee and immigrant men face isolation, loneliness, discrimination and intolerance of their cultural practices, all of which can contribute to their ill-health. In the study I conducted on violence in refugee families (Rees & Pease, 2007), discrimination was identified as a serious problem or a very serious problem by 27.5% of the male sample. Many of the men described experiences of being verbally assaulted. The western media has contributed to the creation of negative images of Muslim people and this has undoubtedly had a profound impact on refugees and their capacity to experience social inclusion. We also know that racism and discrimination have a negative effect on physical and mental health (Nazroo, 1997; Mullins & Schulz, 2006; Bentley, 2007). Rich and Ro (2002) identify institutional racism as a major factor shaping immigrant and refugee men's health and their access to high standard healthcare.

## Gender issues facing immigrant and refugee men

The meanings associated with manhood and masculinity within Australian society further complicate the health of immigrant and refugee men. My research with immigrant and refugee men has illustrated that changes in identity, and shifts in gender roles, have a major impact on these men's health. In my interviews with refugee and immigrant men, I found views expressed by men that women and children had more rights than they did. As men lost some of the status they had experienced in their home country, they tended to blame women for demanding equality from them in their relationships (Pease, 2006b). In the life history study of immigrant and refugee men referred to earlier, the following comment from a man from East Africa summed up the views of a lot of the men interviewed.

> The man is the head of the house . . . There are things that the men are entitled to say and do. African women respect that. When you come to this country, I think you find it doesn't work.

A man from Southern Africa expressed a similar view:

> A perfect partner is someone who . . . is willing to make it possible for me to be head of the family. As I always say, you can't have two lions in the same den. It doesn't work. I mean you come home from work, where somebody is your boss, so you get harassed the whole day. You don't want to come home where there is another boss to boss you around the whole day. I mean you will never win.

Migration thus has an impact on men's status and authority within family life and in the wider community. Men's authority is additionally undermined because of a change in their public status, with men being forced to take up employment well below their qualifications. At the same time though, this reinforced the importance of employment in their sense of self, as the following comments illustrate:

> I prefer to be in Kenya. That's for sure . . . There are many things that I can do back home that I can't do here. There's respect back at home.

*In Australia, I completely lost authority in my home. I had to ask . . . I was highly respected where I come from (Kenya) . . . and to drop from there to here . . . was a very big shock.*

*So overnight from gallivanting around Havana, I had to be stuck in my house 24 hours a day . . . Cleaning the dishes and cooking . . . I had to change my whole background, my whole identity.*

*It would be better to be a man in Bolivia . . . There's a saying in Bolivia. That it's better to be the head of a mouse than the tail of a lion. In Bolivia at least, I would be the head of a mouse. Here, I am pretty close to being the tail of a lion.*

The enactment of masculinity was closely associated with the 'provider role' in all of the home countries of the participants in my research. The issue of being the sole provider was central to all of these men's sense of identity. As such, when they migrate, men experience a threat to their ability to maintain the provider role and they experience challenges to their authority in the family. At the same time, they endeavour to maintain their traditional conception of masculinity and manhood in the face of the challenges they experience. The results of this study suggest that men experience significant marginalisation within Australian culture and have difficulties contending with an increase in the status of women.

Byrne's (2006) work has also reinforced this point, suggesting that one of the most important influences on refugee men's mental health is their loss of identity resulting from a loss of traditional male roles and their perception that women and children gain increased rights. He argues that the problems refugee men face in reconstructing their identity poses major health risks for them. Coello and Aroche (1998) argue that loss of identity associated with resettlement has more of an influence on refugee men's mental health than domestic violence, substance abuse, unemployment and family breakdown.

Coello and Aroche (1998) acknowledge that there are also 'indirect refugee men's health issues' where men's experiences have an impact on the health of others, especially in relation to marital and family relationships. One of the key issues that came out of my research with immigrant and refugee men was that the changes in gender roles and expectations generated high levels of family conflict which in some instances led to domestic violence (Rees & Pease, 2007). While refugee men are oppressed by racial stratification and their marginalised status, they nevertheless have gendered power over refugee women.

Much like those seen in relation to black men in the US (Mutua 2006), one response to the issues facing refugee men is to suggest improvements in their access to patriarchal privileges. Byrne (2006), for example, is concerned that traditional male values and roles are often portrayed as oppressing women and that there is an overconcern with the impact of men's behaviour on women's health and women's rights. In fact, naming patriarchy, dominant masculinity and men's violence as issues that need to be addressed in men's health promotion has invoked a charge by some men's health writers as advocating a 'deficiency syndrome' or a 'deficit' approach to men's health (McDonald et al., 2000). McDonald et al. (2000) emphasise the importance of focusing on what they see as the positive in 'maleness' and male culture. However, in promoting a positive language around 'male energy' and the 'male sex drive' and establishing a foundation that being male is good (McDonald et al., 2000), they demonstrate an essentialist understanding of men's health issues.

In applying this notion to refugee men's health issues, Byrne (2006, p.5) advocates a strength-based approach that provides refugee men 'with more opportunities to experience the positive aspects of traditional masculinity', including men's preoccupation with physical prowess and competition. The strength-based approach is a model of social work theory and practice developed by Saleeby (2002) which emphasises the capacities and strengths of clients. It has been criticised for failing to acknowledge the structural barriers that clients face and by placing too much responsibility on individuals to bring about change (Healy, 2005).

I would argue further that the strengths-based approach does not address situations where people are situated in power relationships with others. In this case, no consideration was given to what a positive approach to male culture might mean for refugee women. There is a danger that by strongly asserting manhood, the patriarchal legacies will remain unquestioned. Strength-based approaches to men's health that do not address gender justice within immigrant and refugee communities are likely to foster a patriarchal manhood that stands above women, rather than standing beside them as equals.

## Conclusion

The argument of this chapter is that there is an intersection between gender, class, ethnicity and race that produces specific health issues for immigrant and refugee men.[3] Refugee men and some immigrant men,

---

[3] I am conscious that I have not explored the issues facing gay, bisexual and transgendered immigrant and refuge men in this chapter.

depending upon their class and race, face significant challenges during settlement. When they arrive, they face unemployment, poverty and racism and have to deal with intergenerational conflict, family breakdown and loss of status and power. Given that many of these groups face racial discrimination, residential segregation and poverty, the social causes of the health issues facing immigrant and refugee men seems overwhelmingly persuasive.

The implications of the approach advocated here is that many aspects of the health status of marginalised men are shaped more by class, race, ethnicity and immigrant/refugee status than by sex or gender. Furthermore, there is overwhelming evidence that the differences between the health of non-white and white men are more related to social factors than race or ethnicity per se (Rich & Ro, 2002). Thus to improve the health of immigrant and refugee men, there will need to be changes in unemployment, housing conditions, institutionalised racism (Kirby & Kirby, 1999) and patriarchal gender relations, rather than strength-based approaches to men's health promotion that are informed by essentialist and sex role theories of masculinity.

## References

Allen, J. (2002) Men interminably in crisis: historians on masculinity, sexual boundaries and manhood. *Radical History Review*, **82**, 191–207.

Barker, G. (2005) *Dying to Be Men: Youth, Masculinity and Social Exclusion*. London: Routledge.

Bentley, M. (2007) *A Primary Health Care Approach to Men's Health in Community Health Settings: 'It's Just Better Practice'*. Adelaide: Flinders University.

Bhopal, R. (2007) *Ethnicity, Race and Health in Multicultural Societies: Foundations for Better Epidemiology, Public Health and Health Care*. New York: Oxford University Press.

Brown, T. (2003) Critical race theory speaks to the sociology of mental health: mental health problems produced by racial stratification. *Journal of Health and Social Behaviour*, **44**(3), 292–301.

Bushra, J. (2000) Gender and forced migration: Editorial. *Forced Migration*, **9**(Dec), 1–7.

Byrne, M. (2006) *The Other Half: Refugee Men's Health*. Sydney: New South Wales Refugee Men's Health Service.

Chambers, D. (1989) *Contemporary problems in the study of masculinities: a comparison between Australia and Britain*. Paper presented at the Australian Sociological Association Conference, La Trobe University, Melbourne.

Coello, M. & Aroche, J. (1998) Refugee men's health. In: *Health and Human Rights: Refugee Health: An Issue for Action – First National Symposium* (eds M. Cunningham, E. Harris & E. Comino). NSW, Australia: Warwick Farm.

Collier, R. (1998) *Masculinities, Crime and Criminology*. London: Sage Publications.

Connell, R.W. (1987) *Gender and Power: Society, the Person and Sexual Politics.* Cambridge: Polity Press.

Connell, R.W. (1995) *Masculinities.* Sydney: Allen & Unwin.

Connell, R.W. (2000) *The Men and the Boys.* Sydney: Allen & Unwin.

Connell, R.W. & Messerschmidt, J. (2005) Hegemonic masculinity: rethinking the concept. *Gender and Society,* **19**(6), 829–859.

Courtenay, W. (2002) A global perspective on men's health: an editorial. *International Journal of Men's Health,* **1**(1), 1–13.

Courtenay, W., McCreary, D. & Merighi, J. (2002) Gender and ethnic differences in health beliefs and behaviours. *Journal of Health Psychology,* **7**(3), 219–231.

Coyle, A. & Morgan-Sykes, C. (1998) Troubled men and threatening women: the construction of crisis in male mental health. *Feminism and Psychology,* **8**(3), 263–284.

Daniels, J. & Schulz, A. (2006) Constructing whiteness in health disparities research. In: *Gender, Race, Class and Health: Intersectional Perspectives* (eds A. Schulz & L. Mullins). San Francisco: Jossey-Bass.

Donaldson, M. (1993) What is hegemonic masculinity? *Theory and Society,* **32**, 643–657.

Doyal, L. (2002) Gender equity in health: debates and dilemmas. In: *Gender, Health and Healing: The Public-Private Divide* (eds G. Bendelow, M. Carpenter, C. Vautier & S. Williams), pp.183–197. New York: Routledge.

Eisler, R. & Herson, M. (1999) *Handbook of Gender, Culture and Health.* Mahwah, NJ: Lawrence Erlbaum.

Ferguson, H. (2001) Men and masculinities in late modern Ireland. In: *A Man's World? Changing Men's Practices in a Globalized World* (eds B. Pease & K. Pringle), pp.118–134. London: Zed Books.

Fletcher, R. (1995) *An Introduction to the New Men's Health.* Newcastle, Australia: Men's Health Project.

Healy, K. (2005) *Social Work Theories in Context: Creating Frameworks for Practice.* Basingstoke, UK: Palgrave Macmillan.

Heartfield, J. (2002) There is no masculinity crisis. *Genders,* **35**, 1–14.

Horrocks, R. (1994) *Masculinity in Crisis.* London: St Martin's Press.

Iacuone, D. (2005) 'Real men are tough guys': hegemonic masculinity and safety in the construction industry. *Journal of Men's Studies,* **13**(2), 247–266.

Jefferson, T. (1994) Theorizing masculine subjectivity. In: *Just Boys Doing Business? Men, Masculinities and Crime* (eds T. Newburn & E. Stanko), pp.10–31. London: Routledge.

Jones, A. (2006) *Men of the Global South.* London: Zed Books.

Jones-Correa, M. (2000) Different paths: gender, immigration and political participation. In: *Gender and Migration* (eds K. Willis & B. Yeoh). Cheltenham, UK: Edward Elgar.

Kaytura, F., Moy, E., Kang, M., Patel, M. & Chesley, F. (2005) Variation in the quality of men's health care by race/ethnicity and social class. *Medical Care,* **43**(3), 72–81.

Kennedy, S. & McDonald, J. (2006) Immigrant mental health and unemployment. *The Economic Record,* **82**(259), 445–459.

Kirby, R. & Kirby, M. (1999) Men's health: closing the gender gap. In: *Men's Health* (eds R. Kirby, M. Kirby and R. Farah). Oxford: Isis Medical Media.

Lorber, J. & Moore, L. (2002) *Gender and the Social Construction of Illness.* Lanham, MD: Rowman & Littlefield.

Luck, M., Bamford, M. & Williamson, P. (2000) *Men's Health: Perspectives, Diversity and Paradox*. Oxford: Blackwell.

Luke, A. (1997) Representing and reconstructing Asian masculinities: this is not a movie review. *Social Alternatives*, **16**(3), 32–34.

Majors, R. (1989) Cool pose: the proud signature of Black survival. In: *Men's Lives* (eds M. Kimmel & M. Messner), pp.83–87. New York: Macmillan.

McCoy, B. (2004) *Kanyirninpa: health, masculinity and the wellbeing of desert men*. PhD thesis, Centre for the Study of Health and Society, University of Melbourne.

McDonald, J., McDermott, M., Brown, A. & Sliwak, G. (2000) *A salutogenic approach to men's health: challenging the sterotypes*. Paper presented at the 12 National Health Promotion Conference, Melbourne, 30 October–2 November.

McDowell, L. (2000) The trouble with men?: Young people, gender transformations and the crisis of masculinity. *International Journal of Urban and Regional Research*, **24**(1), 201–209.

Messner, M. (1997) *Politics of Masculinities: Men in Movements*. Thousand Oaks, CA: Sage Publications.

Mullins, L. & Schulz, A. (2006) Intersectionality and health: an introduction. In: *Gender, Race, Class and Health: Intersectional Approaches* (eds A. Schulz & L. Mullins), pp.3–20. San Francisco: Jossey-Bass.

Mutua, A. (2006) Introduction: mapping the contours of progressive masculinities. In: *Progressive Black Masculinities* (ed. A.D. Mutua), pp.xi–xxviii. New York: Routledge.

Nazroo, J. (1997) *The Health of Britain's Ethnic Minorities*. London: Policy Studies Institute.

Pease, B. (1999) The politics of men's health promotion. *Just Policy*, **15**, 29–35.

Pease, B. (2002) *Men and Gender Relations*. Melbourne: Tertiary Press.

Pease, B. (2004) Decentring white men: critical reflections on masculinity and white studies. In: *Whitening Race: Essays in Social and Cultural Criticism* (ed. A. Moreton-Robinson), pp.119–130. Canberra: Aboriginal Studies Press.

Pease, B. (2006a) Governing men and boys in public policy in Australia. In: *Analysing Social Policy: A Governmental Approach* (G. Marston & C. McDonald), pp.127–144. Cheltenham, UK: Edward Elgar.

Pease, B. (2006b) Australia: masculine migrations. In: *Men of the Global South: A Reader* (ed. A. Jones), pp.343–348. London: Zed Books.

Poynting, S., Noble, G. & Tabar, P. (1998) 'If anybody calls me a wog, they wouldn't be speaking to me alone': protest masculinity and Lebanese youth in Western Sydney. *Journal of Interdisciplinary Gender Studies*, **3**(2), 76–94.

Rees, S. & Pease, B. (2007) Domestic violence in refugee families in Australia: rethinking settlement policy and practice. *Journal of Immigrant and Refugee Studies*, **5**(2), 1–19.

Rich, J. & Ro, M. (2002) *A Poor Man's Plight: Uncovering the Disparity on Men's Health*. Bottle Creek, MI: Kellogg Foundation.

Riska, E. (2006) *Masculinity and Men's Health: Coronary Heart Disease in Medical and Public Discourse*. Lanham, MD: Rowman & Littlefield.

Sabo, D. (1999) *Understanding men's health: a relational and gender sensitive approach*. Paper presented at the Global Health Equity project on Gender and Health Equity, Harvard Center for Population and Development Studies, New York.

Sabo, D. (2005) The study of masculinities and men's health: an overview. In: *Handbook of Studies on Men and Masculinities* (eds M. Kimmel, J. Hearn & R.W. Connell), pp.326–352. Thousand Oaks, CA: Sage Publications.

Sabo, D. & Gordon, D.F. (1995) Rethinking men's health and illness. In: *Men's Health and Illness: Gender, Power, and the Body* (eds D. Sabo & F. Gordon), pp.1–22. Newbury Park, CA: Sage Publications.

Saleeby, D. (2002) *The Strengths Perspective in Social Work.* Boston, MA: Allyn & Bacon.

Sayad, A. (1999) *The Suffering of the Immigrant.* Cambridge: Polity Press.

Schofield, T. (2004) *Boutique Health? Gender and Equity in Health Policy.* Australian Health Policy Institute, Commissioned Paper Series, University of Sydney.

Schofield, T., Connell, R.W., Walker, L., Wood, J. & Butland, D. (2000) Understanding men's health and illness: a gender relations approach to policy, research and practice. *Journal of American College Health*, **48**, 247–256.

Seidler, V. (2006) *Young Men and Masculinities: Global Cultures and Intimate Lives.* London: Zed Books.

Smedley, B., Stith, A. & Neslon, A. (2004) *Unequal Treatment: Confronting Racial and Ethnic Disparities in Health Care.* Washington, DC: National Academies Press.

Stanistreet, D. (2005) Constructions of marginalized masculinities among young men who die through opiate use. *International Journal of Men's Health*, **4**(3), 243–266.

Steel, Z., Silove, D., Phan, T. & Bauman, A. (2002) Long-term effect of psychological trauma on the mental health of Vietnamese refugees resettled in Australia: a population-based study. *Lancet*, **360**(9339), 1056–1062.

Syme, S. & Berkman, L. (1990) Social class, susceptibility and sickness. In: *The Sociology of Health and Illness* (eds P. Conrad & R. Kern), pp.24–30. New York: St Martin's Press.

Tashiro, C. (2005) Health disparities in the context of mixed race: challenging the ideology of race. *Advances in Nursing Science*, **28**(3), 203–211.

Traister, B. (2000) Academic viagra: the rise of American masculinity studies. *American Quarterly*, **52**(2), 274–304.

Wadham, B. (2001) Global men's health and the crisis of western masculinity. In: *A Man's World? Changing Men's Practices in a Globalized World* (eds B. Pease & K. Pringle), pp.69–82. London: Zed Books.

Watson, S. (2000) Foucault and the study of social policy. In: *Rethinking Social Policy* (eds G. Lewis, S. Gewitz & J. Clarke), pp.66–77. London: Sage Publications.

Weber, L. (2006) Reconstructing the landscape of health disparities research: promoting dialogue and collaboration between feminist intersectional and biomedical paradigms. In: *Gender, Race, Class and Health: Intersectional Perspectives* (eds A. Schulz & L. Mullins), pp.21–59. San Francisco: Jossey-Bass.

Weber, L. & Para-Medina, D. (2003) Intersectionality and women's health: charting a path to eliminating health disparities. In: *Gender Perspectives on Health and Medicine: Key Themes, Advances in Gender Research* , Vol 7 (eds M.T. Segal & V. Demos), pp.181–230. Oxford: Elsevier.

White, R. (2002) Social and political aspects of men's health. *Health: An Interdisciplinary Journal for the Study of Health, Illness and Medicine*, **6**(3), 267–285.

Whitehead, S. (2002) *Men and Masculinities: Key Themes and New Directions.* Cambridge: Polity Press.

Wilkinson, R. (1996) *Unhealthy Societies: The Afflictions of Inequality.* London: Routledge.

Willis, D. & Porche, D. (2006) Envisaging and advancing marginalized men's health disparities scholarship: the marginality-cultural competence integrative framework. *Issues in Mental Health Nursing,* **27**, 425–442.

Willis, K. & Yeoh, B. (2000) *Gender and Migration.* Cheltingham, UK: Edward Elgar.

Woodward, A., Mathews, C. & Tobias, M. (2001) Migrants, money and margarine: possible explanations for Australian–New Zealand mortality differences. In: *The Social Origins of Health and Well-being* (eds R. Eckersley, J. Dixon & B. Douglas), pp.114–128. Cambridge: Cambridge University Press.

# Chapter 10

# FUTURE RESEARCH AGENDA IN MEN'S HEALTH

Alan Petersen

## Introduction

A major challenge confronting those who seek to understand and improve men's health is developing appropriate frameworks for making sense of and appropriately responding to the diverse and rapidly accumulating research data in this field. Some questions that arise include: what significance should be attributed to different kinds of research evidence (e.g. genetic, psychological, sociological)? To what extent do reported differences between men and women in mental and physical health status reflect differences in patterns of usage of healthcare services or methods of reporting? Do attempts to measure difference actually help construct or reinforce difference? Insofar as health outcomes can be shown to be generated by conditions that are alterable, what changes are required and how might they be implemented? Perhaps most importantly, how do we know that the questions posed by researchers are the 'right' ones?

As I argue in this chapter, a number of the assumptions and perspectives that have guided research thus far are likely to limit rather than advance understanding of and action on men's health by narrowing the field of focus. Further, if one is to develop a research agenda that has real impact on the lives of men and their partners and families it is essential first to articulate these assumptions and perspectives and to be aware of how they shape thinking and action. While the recent focus on men's health matters is welcome, in the absence of reflection on the guiding assumptions of the field and greater understanding of their predisposing historical and social contexts, there is the danger that research will reinforce rather than change the conditions that lead to illness, injury and premature death among men. The chapter outlines some of the major assumptions and perspectives and offers some suggestions as to how the research agenda may be fruitfully advanced.

## Some guiding assumptions in research

Many assumptions about men, masculinities and health are essentialist. Essentialism, or belief in an invariable essence, whether of sex/gender, 'race', or class, or indeed any attribute, has been a recurring feature of modern western thought (Sayer, 1997). In particular, the belief that there is an essential or 'natural' difference between men and women in reasoning, temperament, outlook and behaviours that may affect their physical, psychological and emotional wellbeing, has proved difficult to dispel. The language and metaphors of difference are deeply embedded within contemporary culture, circulating widely via diverse media, including popular books such as Pease and Pease's *Why Men Don't Listen and Women Can't Read Maps* (2001), Gray's *Men Are From Mars, Women are From Venus* (1992) and Moir and Moir's *Why Men Don't Iron* (1998). For example, the notion of the 'hysterical woman', which sees a woman's mental wellbeing as linked to her reproductive system, has a long historical lineage (see Ehrenreich and English, 1979). Similarly, the discourse of the male sex drive, which suggests that men's sexuality is 'driven' by a biological imperative (Hollway, 1984), has had an enduring influence on thinking about sexuality and gender in the modern western world. Despite considerable 'second-wave' and later feminist efforts to debunk the notion of 'biology-as-destiny' by showing the historical and cross-cultural variability of constructions of masculinity and femininity, the notion that men and women are 'in essence' 'made-up' and think differently, but in ways that are complementary, continues to shape policy and action at many levels, including in relation to men's health. This two-sex/two-gender model is a product of Enlightenment thinking and of efforts to limit women's involvement in the public sphere, which involved the considerable assistance of philosophers and anatomists (Lloyd, 1984; Laqueur, 1990; Schiebinger, 1993).

Scientists, social scientists, feminists and 'pro-feminist' male scholars and activists have often uncritically adopted and contributed to the development of theories of 'essential' difference in their writings. Theories of the psychology of sex differences and of psychoanalysis (e.g. Nancy Chodorow's *The Reproduction of Mothering* (1978) and Carol Gilligan's *In a Different Voice* (1982)) have been especially influential, resonating with broadly shared views on male/female propensities, outlooks and behaviours. Theories of differences in men's and women's propensity to engage in aggressive behaviour, with men being seen as 'naturally more aggressive', for example, has been explained through the history of psychology as variously due to instinct differences, genetic differences and other innate differences. This neglects historical and cross-cultural variations in definitions of behaviours seen as appropriate for males and females and suggests that aggressive behaviour is unalterable (Petersen, 1997). The difficulty of breaking with essentialism is hardly surprising given its history and its compatibility with dominant interests and frameworks. Gender essentialism is historically entrenched in law, for example in the concept of the 'reasonable man' which provides a basis for making judgements about appropriate human conduct and is used in evidence submitted in cases involving men's violence (Naffine, 1987, 1995).

There is a need for greater reflection on the implications of assumptions about 'essential' differences and how these may be perpetuated through the pursuit of particular policies and research questions and reliance on certain kinds of evidence. One question which frequently arises in the context of men's health is: how may research findings showing differences in men's and women's mortality or morbidity be evaluated and how should policy-makers respond? Some conditions or behaviours that are claimed to be inherent to men ('hard-wired') by virtue of their biology (e.g. 'testosterone-fuelled' violence, promiscuous sexual behaviour) can be shown (e.g. by other, historical and cross-cultural evidence) to be shaped by social expectations and environments. While there may be a long history of differences between men and women in patterns of illness and behaviour, this does not mean that the differences are biologically based and immutable. To suggest that a difference is 'essential' or 'natural' implies that it is fixed for all time and, in relation to certain problematic behaviours, justified. For example, men's violent behaviour and unwillingness to take equal responsibility for the care of children and the elderly and sick may be, and sometimes has been, excused as a 'fact of nature'. Sociobiology and evolutionary psychology have often provided the explanatory frameworks in discussions about sex-based differences. These theories draw extensively on evidence from studies of primates and other animals, as well as studies from criminal statistics, to support arguments that differences have evolved due to their adaptive value for the species (Nelkin, 2000). Adherence to such frameworks may divert attention from much-needed social changes that affect the lives and relationships of both women and men. As emphasised in the previous chapters which provide key substantive examples, researchers need to reject essentialist thinking if they are to advance men's health without reinforcing existing inequalities.

## Dualistic thought

This discursive practice of reifying gender difference is closely linked to and reliant on another taken-for-granted premise; namely, that the world

is 'naturally' characterised by, and is most fruitfully understood by reference to, oppositional pairs or dualisms. Dualisms pertain to many dimensions of the physical and social world: man/woman, masculine/feminine,
sex/gender, heterosexual/homosexual, self/other, nature/culture, subject/
object, local/global, public/private, pure/impure, mind/body and health/
illness. Each of these dichotomies relies on other dichotomies which are
very often positively or negatively connoted. For example, in contemporary
western cultures, 'man' and 'masculine' are coded heterosexual, which is
valued as the 'normal', healthy self and opposed to the 'abnormal', pathologised other, the homosexual. Maintaining the 'purity' of heterosexual masculinity is seen to involve the denial, exclusion or 'treatment' of the
'impure' homosexual other, who is seen to present the ever-present danger
of polluting identity and is thus to be feared and despised. Early HIV/AIDS
policies were premised on this dualistic distinction which had a significant
deleterious impact on the lives of homosexual men, who were often blamed
and persecuted for 'spreading illness', which in many cases originated with
avowedly heterosexual men who were having sex with other men (Jagose,
1996). By focusing on (pathologised) *identities* rather than *acts*, AIDS education policy often failed to promote safe-sex messages to actual 'at risk'
groups (Jagose, 1996). Thinking about sexualities as fluid rather than as
fixed (e.g. by genes) is likely to prove challenging for many self-identified
heterosexual men, but the adoption of a more dynamic conception of masculine sexuality would contribute towards the development of a more
tolerant society and men's greater understanding of their own sexuality
and health. Dualist thought works against seeing problems 'holistically':
the links between gay men's health and heterosexual men's health; the
inextricable connection between physical health and psychological and
emotional wellbeing; the interdependence of men's health and women's
health, and so on.

One of the important contributions of recent research on men and masculinities, as illustrated in the chapters of this book, has been to unsettle
the crude dualism of masculine/feminine. The pluralised 'masculinities'
emphasises the heterogeneous character of men's lives which are differentiated according to class, ethnicity, age, sexuality, and place of residence.
Raewyn Connell (1995) has referred to a hierarchy of masculinities, with
white, western heterosexual men occupying the dominant position. The
acknowledgement of this heterogeneity in men's situations and experiences unsettles simplistic, dualistic conceptions of gender differences in
health, illness and mortality. Differences between men in behaviours,
experiences and health outcomes, in some contexts, may be as substantial
or be more significant than differences between men and women. Just as
white western feminists' core concepts such as 'women' and universal

sisterhood were challenged by the perspectives of black women and women from the developing world (Grant, 1993), the frameworks of (mostly) white male self-identified heterosexual writers who write about 'men's experiences' (including their health and illness) as though they were homogenous are being challenged by the growing evidence produced about and by men and women from minority ethnic, religious and gay communities. However, while it is important to acknowledge the multiplicity of masculinities, one should not overlook the significance of the discourses, institutions and practices that tend to work in favour of the dominance of men *in general*.

## The dominance of biomedical conceptions of health

A notable institution in this respect is that of biomedicine which, as many feminists have argued, exhibits a gender bias in its discourses and practices. Anatomy, a core discipline in medical education, is gendered in its conceptualisation of male/female biophysical difference, in its history of teaching and research, and in its professional membership (Petersen & Regan de Bere, 2006). Biomedicine is characterised by its reductive, positivist approach to health and illness. Within the biomedical worldview, mind and body are seen as separable: the focus is resolutely on the body, which tends to be treated without reference to the person and their emotions. This so-called Cartesian dualism involves reductionism in that the person is reduced to their body, which is viewed as a machine in need of repair (and increasingly, improvement) with the assistance of the (mostly male) expert medical practitioner (Petersen, 2007, pp.105–10). It reinforces an instrumental view of the body, as subject to rational control by the mind, which is arguably implicated in a number of body-related problems, such as anorexia, bulimia and dangerous levels of exercising and other forms of body management (Petersen 2007: 110–112). The biomedical worldview allows little tolerance for imperfection and uncertainty in relation to diagnosis and treatment. Medicine promises bodily perfection and the resolution of problems once and for all.

In the context of many complementary and alternative medicines (CAMs), on the other hand, it is generally accepted that the mind and body are inseparable and that healing requires attention to the 'whole person', including their emotional life and physical and social environment, and that health is a process requiring ongoing work on the self. This is not to say that CAMs are not without their own shortcomings (see Tovey et al., 2004; Petersen, 2007). However, their growing popularity does point to growing recognition of significant problems with the state of biomedicine including its gender biases. Significantly, women are more likely to turn to complementary and alternative therapies than men (Eisenberg et al., 1998; Ni et al., 2002; Ong & Banks, 2003), a fact that may be related to medicine's long history of objectifying women's bodies and its failure to deal adequately with many of the particular health problems that women encounter. The limits of biomedical reductionism have become apparent in relation to treating illness, leading as it does to the objectification of the patient and an over-reliance on often-dangerous drugs and invasive surgical procedures that may adversely affect the health of men and women. Increasingly, however, it is recognised that men's bodies and men's health, too, are subject to medicalisation, though to a different extent and in different ways (see Rosenfeld & Faircloth, 2006).

The increasing emphasis on genetic explanations in medicine and more generally arguably reinforces the idea that apparent differences between men and women are 'hard-wired' or 'essential' differences. Genetic explanations focus attention on supposed 'defects' in our make-ups and behaviours and on 'quick fix' 'treatments', which deny the considerable historical and cross-cultural variability in conceptions of normality and the limits in the ability of biomedicine to resolve problems that have a complex aetiology. These biases and orientations are deeply entrenched in history and shape contemporary cultural practices including scientific research, for example on genetic-based differences of sex and sexual orientation (see Petersen, 1999), and the teaching and learning of human anatomy in medical education (Petersen & Regan de Bere, 2006). The preoccupation with genetics in medicine has led to the search for 'personalised' drugs; that is, drugs that are 'tailored' to the individual, to the neglect of action on the social and environmental conditions that arguably have a profound impact on the individual's state of health. Genetics has also been used to explain and justify differences between men and women in career prospects and life chances (Petersen, 1999). The Darwinian theory of evolutionary selection underlying this genetic essentialism suggests that differences are adaptive and that those who survive and thrive (i.e. males) are inherently strong, while those who are prone to sickness and incapacity (i.e. females) are weak and ill-adapted to the demands of work and public life.

There is a need to broaden the conception of health to include reference to the complex, interrelated range of issues that may affect men's and women's wellbeing, including an entrenched division of paid and unpaid labour, economic and social inequalities, interpersonal violence and environmental degradation. A broadened, public health approach locates discrete problems that are identified in the clinic, the criminal justice system, and other settings, within a sociocultural and politicoeconomic context. This approach is broadly in line with the ideals of the so-called 'new public health'. While such an approach as developed thus far has not been without its limitations and unacknowledged implications (see Petersen & Lupton, 1996), it does at least recognise the need to view problems of health and illness as amenable to policy intervention and as subject to complementary intervention on a number of fronts. Within a public health framework, premature death among young men due to, for example, suicide, reckless driving, alcohol and drug abuse, and pursuit in high-risk sports and leisure activities may each call for a range of actions at a number of levels: sociocultural (e.g. changing the norms that strongly link auto-mobility with masculinity; see Hård & Jamison, 2005), legislative (e.g. laws governing the conditions of drinking, vehicle licensing requirements) and behavioural (e.g. improved systems of family support).

## Developing new perspectives on men's health and illness

What the foregoing emphasises is the need to develop new perspectives on men's health and illness. Researchers in the field of men and masculinities studies in general, and men's health in particular, often remain wedded to crude, modernist conceptions of society and fail to engage with recent theoretical debates within feminism and social science about the workings of politics and power in contemporary societies. The adherence to 'totalising' theories and the search for universal truths works against the exploration of new modes of ('rhizomatic') thought and existence (Deleuze & Guattari, 1987). The lingering influence of 'second-wave' feminism is notable in much research – in references to all-pervasive patriarchy, outdated conceptions of 'oppression', 'consciousness-raising', and so on. Given how frequently men's studies scholars claim to be pro-feminist, anti-racist and non-homophobic, it is surprising how often in their research and writings they fail to engage with the many strands of thought that characterise contemporary feminism, anti-racist/post-colonial studies, and gay and lesbian scholarship (Petersen, 2003). Postmodern and post-structural (including Foucauldian) scholarship, eco-feminism, post-colonial and Developing World studies, and gay and lesbian scholarship have much to contribute to thinking about men's health, as they do about other aspects of men's lives. Each of these different fields presents a somewhat different 'take' on the workings of power and on the relationship between power and knowledge. Michel Foucault's concepts of 'bio-politics' and 'practices of the self' (Foucault, 1980, 1985, 1986), for example, may find useful application in this field, raising new questions about issues such as the relationship between social norms and expectations and individual behaviours, and the scope for developing new, more caring practices of the self.

In particular, there is need for more historically informed research and genealogical work along the lines proposed by Foucault and his followers which challenges the self-evidence of our current ways of thinking and action; for example, in relation to mental illness and depression, self-care and risk-taking (e.g. McCallum, 1997; Nettleton, 1997; Petersen, 1997). Researchers rely heavily on certain methodologies, notably surveys, interviews and focus groups, and neglect historical, critical deconstructive approaches, which reflects the close linking of academic research to narrow policy agendas and the pursuit of 'quick fixes' to what are complex problems. A more critical, historically oriented and theoretically informed approach to men's health would give acknowledgment to the often powerful interests underlying specific definitions of men's health problems; for example, as diseases requiring expensive and often dangerous drugs. It would be oriented to confronting those interests (e.g. pharmaceutical companies) that target their products (e.g. impotence drugs; see Loe, 2004) and services to particular groups of men, and to changing those conditions (e.g. work environments; see Waldron, 1995) that predispose to illness, disability and premature death.

An approach such as that outlined would also seek to provide deeper insight into the gendering of risk, and particularly why in many contemporary societies there has come to be a close link between certain constructions of masculinity and men's engagement in extremely risky activities. This includes excessive alcohol consumption and other drug-taking and participation in dangerous sports and leisure activities that very often lead to illness, injury and death. The propensity for young, working-class men in particular to engage in extreme risk-taking pursuits, so-called 'edge-work' (Lyng, 2005), is little understood at present yet begs for analysis. This calls for consideration of issues that are generally not addressed within the biomedical framework, such as the experience of economic and social marginalisation, the class-, ethnic and gender-related expectations pertaining to body management (Bourdieu, 1986), and the variable standards of emotional expression for men and women (Stearns, 1993). An exploration of emotionality offers considerable potential for illuminating men's investments in extreme risk-taking and other practices that affect men's health. The sociology of emotions has highlighted the 'emotional labour' involved in certain gender-specific work, such as in the service sector, and how this may affect people's wellbeing. However, research to date has tended to focus almost exclusively on women's experiences, which is not surprising given their greater contribution to the service industry, care in general, and 'sex work' (e.g. Dunscombe & Marsden, 1993, 1996; Hochschild, 1983, 2003). An exploration of the constructions of masculinities and emotional expression and experience has the potential to cast light on such questions as why so many men feel compelled to engage in violent and especially 'risky' activities (Lois, 2005); why they respond as they do to the onset of chronic illness (Charmaz, 1995); why they are more 'successful' than women in their suicide attempts (Canetto, 1995); and how they negotiate the norms regarding 'ideal' body size and shape (Monaghan, 2007).

The proposed research agenda for men's health would not only seek to illuminate the conditions that give rise to and 'normalise' certain practices predisposing to violence, self-injury, illness and premature death, but would also propose workable, long-lasting solutions to problems. The broad public health approach would shift the focus from changing 'men' to changing the discourses, institutions and practices that reinforce certain problematic masculine behaviours. This includes challenging the deeply gendered institutions of the family, work, the law, religion, science and the media. Re-directing research endeavours away from questions of 'difference' to questions of 'sameness' would be a useful start in this direction. Men and women are more similar in respect to their genetic make-up and everyday material needs and experiences than they are different. However, research continues to be preoccupied with questions of difference. As noted, such a perspective is reinforced through popular media that increasingly suggest that identity, including gender identity, is a matter of 'consumer choice' (Petersen, 2004). This serves to divert attention from the social structures and values that shape (although do not determine) individual beliefs and actions.

Rapidly growing disparities in wealth at global and national levels underline the significance of access to economic resources and of power relations for determining people's life chances and wellbeing. Advanced liberal rule, which places emphasis on individuality and 'powers of freedom' (Rose, 1999), while eroding notions of social solidarity and collective action, however, operates to 'naturalise' difference by reinforcing the idea that life chances are simply a matter of chance (e.g. 'faulty' genes) or a consequence of the exercise of 'good' and 'bad' decisions in the free market. There is a need to place questions of power relations and unequal access to the conditions that shape health and wellbeing firmly on the agenda of men's research. Greater recognition needs to be paid to the historical and cross-cultural variability in constructions of gender and in conceptions of the body, health and illness. A rich anthropological and historical scholarship has revealed that conceptions of 'health' and 'illness' and the rules for conduct pertaining to men and women vary considerably through time and across societies and that there is consequently considerable scope for rethinking 'men's health'. A research agenda that takes this as a starting point for enquiries, I believe, will do much to advance the health and wellbeing of both men and women in the future.

# References

Bourdieu, P. (1986) *Distinction: A Social Critique of the Judgement of Taste*. London: Routledge & Kegan Paul.

Canetto, S.S. (1995) Men who survive a suicidal act. In: *Men's Health and Illness: Gender, Power and the Body* (eds D. Sabo & D.F. Gordon), pp.292–304. London: Sage Publications.

Charmaz, K. (1995) Identity dilemmas of chronically ill men. In: *Men's Health and Illness: Gender, Power and the Body* (eds D. Sabo & D.F. Gordon), pp.266–291. London: Sage Publications.

Chodorow, N. (1978) *The Reproduction of Mothering*. Berkeley, CA: University of California Press.

Connell, R.W. (1995) *Masculinities*. Berkeley, CA: University of California Press.

Deleuze, G. & Guattari, F. (1987) *A Thousand Plateaus: Capitalism and Schizophrenia*. Minneapolis, MN: University of Minnesota Press.

Duncombe, J. & Marsden, D. (1993) Love and intimacy: the gender division of emotion and 'emotion work': a neglected aspect of sociological discussion of heterosexual relationships. *Sociology*, **27**(2), 221–241.

Duncombe, J. & Marsden, D. (1996) 'Workaholics' and 'winging women': theorizing intimacy and emotion work: the last frontier of gender inequality. *Sociological Review*, **43**(1), 150–169.

Ehrenreich, B. & English, D. (1979) *For Her Own Good: 150 Years of the Experts' Advice to Women*. New York: Anchor Books.

Eisenberg, D.M., Davis, R.B., Ettner, S.L. et al. (1998) Trends in alternative medicine use in the United States, 1990–1997 results of a follow-up national survey. *Journal of the American Medical Association*, **280**, 1569–1575.

Foucault, M. (1980) *The History of Sexuality: Volume 1: An Introduction*. New York: Vintage Books.

Foucault, M. (1985) *The Use of Pleasure* (translated by R. Hurley). Harmondsworth, UK: Penguin.

Foucault, M. (1986) *The Care of the Self* (translated by R. Hurley). Harmondsworth, UK: Penguin.

Gilligan, C. (1982) *In a Different Voice: Psychological Theory and Women's Development*. Cambridge, MA: Harvard University Press.

Grant, J. (1993) *Fundamental Feminism: Contesting the Core Concepts of Feminist Theory*. London: Routledge.

Gray, J. (1992) *Men Are From Mars, Women Are From Venus: A Practical Guide for Improving Communication and Getting What you Want in your Relationships*. New York: Harper Collins.

Hård, M. & Jamison, A. (2005) *Hubris and Hybrids: A Cultural History of Technology and Society*. New York; London: Routledge.

Hochschild, A.R. (1983) *The Managed Heart: The Commercialization of Human Feeling*. Berkeley, CA: University of California Press.

Hochschild, A.R. (2003) *The Commercialization of Intimate Life: Notes from Home and Work*. Berkeley, CA: University of California Press.

Hollway, W. (1984) Gender difference and the production of subjectivity. In: *Changing the Subject: Psychology, Social Regulation and Subjectivity* (eds J. Henriques, W. Holloway, C. Urwin, C. Venn & V. Walkerdine), pp.227–263. London; New York: Methuen.

Jagose, A. (1996) *Queer Theory*. Melbourne: Melbourne University Press.

Laqueur, T. (1990) *Making Sex: Body and Gender from the Greeks to Freud*. Cambridge, MA: Harvard University Press.

Lloyd, G. (1984) *The Man of Reason: 'Male' and 'Female' in Western Philosophy*. London: Methuen.

Loe, M. (2004) *The Rise of Viagra: How the Little Blue Pill Changed Sex in America*. New York: New York University Press.

Lois, J. (2005) Gender and emotion management in the stages of edgework. In: *Edgework: The Sociology of Risk-Taking* (ed. S. Lyng), pp.117–152. New York; London: Routledge.

Lyng, S. (2005) *Edgework: The Sociology of Risk-Taking*. New York; London: Routledge.

McCallum, D. (1997) Mental health, criminality and the human sciences. In: *Foucault, Health and Medicine* (eds A. Petersen & R. Bunton), pp.53–73. New York; London: Routledge.

Moir, A. & Moir, B. (1998) *Why Men Don't Iron: The Real Science of Gender Studies*. London: Harper Collins.

Monaghan, L.F. (2007) McDonaldizing men's bodies?: Slimming, associated (ir)rationalities and resistances. *Body & Society*, **13**(2), 67–93.

Naffine, N. (1987) *Female Crime: The Construction of Women in Criminology*. North Sydney: Allen & Unwin.

Naffine, N. (1995) *Gender, Crime and Feminism*. Aldershot, UK: Dartmouth.

Nelkin, D. (2000) Less selfish than sacred? Genes and religious impulse in evolutionary psychology. In: *Alas, Poor Darwin: Arguments Against Evolutionary Psychology* (eds H. Rose & S. Rose), pp.17–32. London: Jonathan Cape.

Nettleton, S. (1997) Governing the risky self: how to become healthy, wealthy and wise. In: *Foucault, Health and Medicine* (eds A. Petersen & R. Bunton), pp.207–222. New York; London: Routledge.

Ni, H., Simile, C. & Hardy, A.M. (2002) Utilization of complementary and alternative medicine by United States adults results from the 1999 National Health Interview Survey. *Medical Care*, **40**, 353–358.

Ong, C-K. & Banks, B. (2003) *Complementary and Alternative Medicine: The Consumer Perspective*. The Prince of Wales Foundation for Integrated Health, p.13. Occasional Paper. Online www.Foundazionericci.it/flex/files/ D.1eOca72fef1b866acb72/ Complementary_and_Alternative_Medicine_the_Consumer_Perspective.pdf. Accessed 21 April 2006.

Pease, A. & Pease, B. (2001) *Why Men Don't Listen and Women Can't Read Maps*. London: Orion Books.

Petersen, A. (1997) Risk, governance and the new public health. In: *Foucault, Health and Medicine* (eds A. Petersen & R. Bunton), pp.189–206. New York; London: Routledge.

Petersen, A. (1999) The portrayal of research into genetic-based differences of sex and sexual orientation: a study of 'popular' science journals, 1980 to 1997. *Journal of Communication Inquiry*, **23**(2), 163–182.

Petersen, A. (2003) Research on men and masculinities: some implications of recent theory for future work. *Men and Masculinities*, **6**(1), 54–69.

Petersen, A. (2004) *Engendering Emotions*. Basingstoke, UK: Palgrave Macmillan.

Petersen, A. (2007) *The Body in Question: A Socio-Cultural Approach*. New York; London: Routledge.

Petersen, A. & Lupton, D. (1996) *The New Public Health: Health and Self in the Age of Risk*. London: Sage Publications.

Petersen, A. & Regan de Bere, S. (2006) Dissecting medicine: gender biases in the discourses and practices of medical anatomy. In: *Medicalized Masculinities* (eds D. Rosenfeld & C.A. Faircloth), pp.112–131. Philadephia, PA: Temple University Press.

Rose, N. (1999) *Powers of Freedom: Reframing Political Thought*. Cambridge: Cambridge University Press.

Rosenfeld, D. & Faircloth, C.A. (2006) *Medicalized Masculinities*. Philadelphia, PA: Temple University Press.

Sayer, A. (1997) Essentialism, social constructionism, and beyond. *Sociological Review*, **45**(3), 453–487.

Schiebinger, L. (1993) *Nature's Body: Gender in the Making of Modern Science*. Cambridge, MA: Harvard University Press.

Stearns, P.N. (1993) Girls, boys, and emotions: redefinitions and historical change. *Journal of American History*, **80**(1), 36–74.

Tovey, P., Easthope, G. & Adams, J. (2004) *The Mainstreaming of Complementary and Alternative Medicine: Studies in Social Context*. London; New York: Routledge.

Waldron, I. (1995) Contributions to changing gender differences in behaviour and social roles to changing gender differences in mortality. In: *Men's Health and Illness: Gender, Power, and the Body* (eds D. Sabo & F. Gordon), pp.22–45. London: Sage Publications.

# INDEX